Natural
Pregnancy

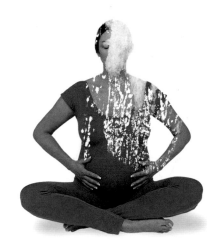

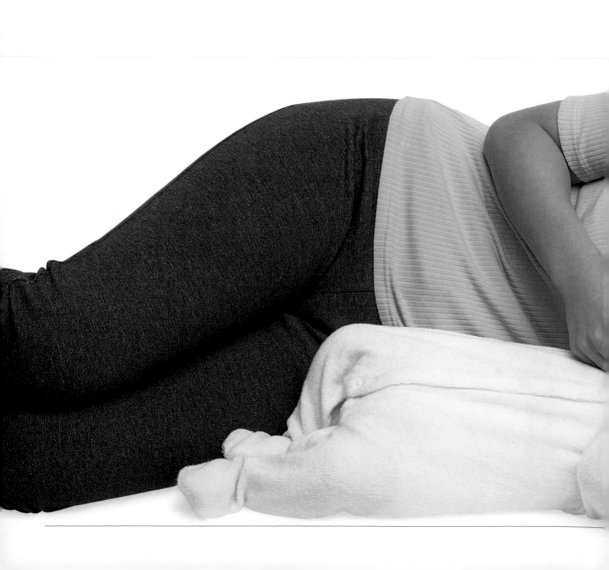

Natural Pregnancy

Zita West

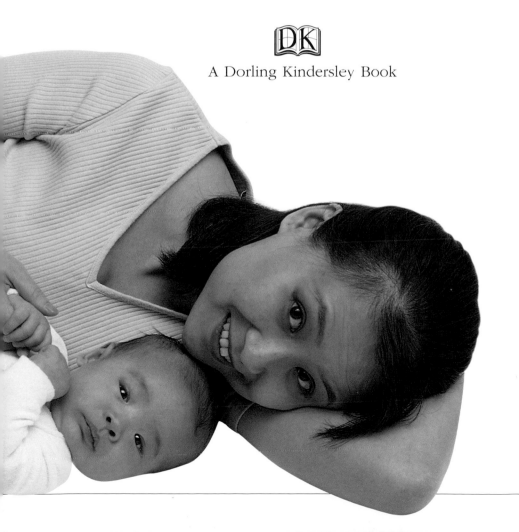

A Dorling Kindersley Book

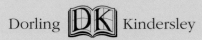

Dorling **DK** Kindersley

London, New York, Munich,
Melbourne, Delhi

Senior Editor Jude Garlick
Senior Art Editor Dawn Terrey
Managing Editor Susannah Marriott
Managing Art Editor Clare Shedden
DTP Designer Conrad van Dyk
Production Controller Maryann Webster
Photographer Andy Crawford

You are strongly advised to consult
a conventional medical practitioner before using
any complementary treatments if you have
symptoms of illness, any diagnosed ailment
or if you are receiving conventional treatment or
medication. Do not cease conventional treatment
or medication without first consulting your
doctor. Always inform your doctor and your
complementary practitioner of any treatments,
medication or remedies that you are
taking or intend to take.

First published in Great Britain in 2001
by Dorling Kindersley Limited
Revised edition published in Great Britain in 2005
by Dorling Kindersley Limited, A Penguin Company
80 Strand, London WC2R ORL

A CIP catalogue record for this book is
available from the British Library.

ISBN 1 4053 0229 1

Reproduced by Colourscan
Printed and bound by Tien Wah Press

See our complete catalogue at
www.dk.com

Contents

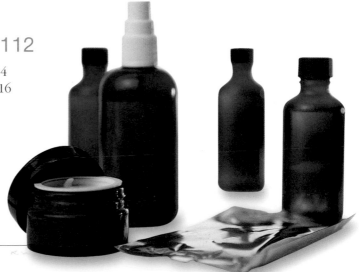

Foreword

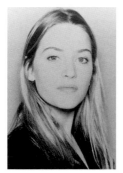

As soon as I found out that I was pregnant, I seemed to be assailed with well-meaning but conflicting advice from every direction. "You should try this", "You shouldn't do that", "You ought to eat this", "You mustn't touch that". All very confusing.

That's why this book became my bible during pregnancy. It really does contain everything you need to know, from information on diet and exercise to tips on how to deal with minor ailments and ways to prepare for labour. Most refreshing of all is that Zita doesn't preach or try to persuade you down a completely "natural" route. She "knows her stuff" but her view is a balanced one which bridges the gap between alternative and orthodox, complementary and conventional.

And she doesn't blind you with science, either. The information is comprehensive, helpful, easy to find and in short digestible chunks (and that's important when you're pregnant!). Reading the book gave me confidence and I'm sure it helped me to cope better during both pregnancy and labour.

Of all the information and advice in the book, I think what I found most fascinating was the section on docosahexaenoic acid (DHA) and how important it is for the baby's developing brain. I rushed straight out to get my own supply. I'm also certain that without Zita's dietary advice and the vitamin supplements I took, I would never have survived filming at 18 weeks.

Before I was pregnant, I thought I knew exactly how I would feel - confident, blooming and sexy – the way celebrities are expected to feel. Not a bit of it! Pregnancy turned out to be one of the hardest things I've ever done, physically, mentally and emotionally. Instead of shining hair and glowing cheeks, the reality was morning sickness, swollen ankles and a bad back, and by the third trimester I felt more like a large red London bus than a film star. Zita's suggestions for alternative remedies made all the difference. The one tip she didn't give was how to cope with hot weather - oh, the joy of sitting in a paddling pool in the garden at 34 weeks, eating ice-cream and wearing the one pair of knickers that still fit!

Kate Winslet

Introduction

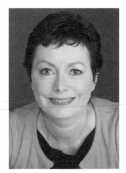

I have worked as a midwife and acupuncturist, both in private practice and within the UK's National Health Service, for many years. I have treated thousands of pregnant women and observed first-hand the growing interest in holistic natural remedies and complementary therapies. During pregnancy, more than at any other time in their lives, women seek natural products, non-invasive treatments and drug-free methods of pain relief that will not harm their babies. So much rests on the healthy, happy outcome of a pregnancy that women want to be involved in their antenatal care. They are unwilling to be passive and "patient". Complementary approaches to antenatal care give a woman choice and help her to regain a feeling of control over her body. Treatments work in harmony with natural rhythms, recognizng the body's innate ability to heal itself. They focus on the person rather than the complaint.

Pregnancy is, after all, a natural physiological event, not an illness. Information, advice and support are what most women are looking for – not diagnosis or cure. Many pregnancy ailments are hard to alleviate conventionally, so orthodox medicine tends to regard them as par for the course. Most mothers-to-be would rather suffer themselves than pop a pill that might have unexpected side effects. But no woman needs to suffer pain or discomfort during pregnancy. Most minor ailments can be relieved by using a combination of complementary therapies. There is a wealth of natural remedies and treatments available – for specific conditions and to enhance general well-being – to ensure that women can enjoy their pregnancies in a state of blooming health.

I hope that this book will provide the reader with useful information – about preconceptual care, development and care in each trimester, preparation for labour, the birth, postnatal care and recommended complementary therapies. With knowledge, practical advice and sensible notes of caution will come the confidence to enjoy your pregnancy and the birth of your baby in good health and with a positive state of mind.

Zita West.

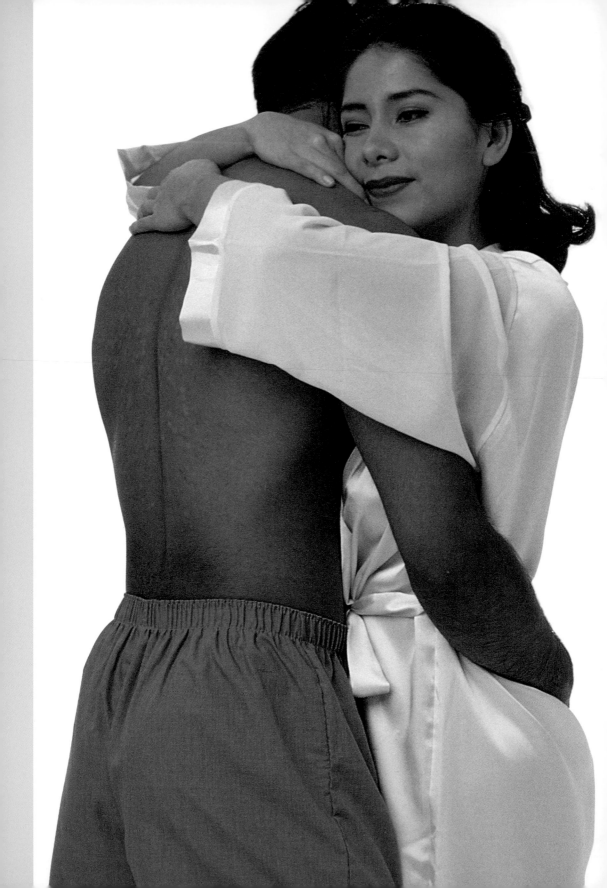

MOST PROSPECTIVE PARENTS these days are unwilling to leave having their babies to chance. More and more couples make plans for conception, pregnancy and birth in advance. Ideally, you and your partner should start to prepare four months before you want to conceive. You should both prepare yourselves physically, nutritionally,

Planning for conception & pregnancy

emotionally and mentally. This section advises you how to improve fertility and fitness prior to conception, and outlines fundamental issues relevant throughout your pregnancy. These include good nutrition, fitness, dealing with illness, your environment, and practicalities that need to be considered, such as antenatal tests.

Getting Fit for Pregnancy

HEALTHY BABIES COME FROM HEALTHY PARENTS. You and your partner should both prepare for pregnancy. Not only will this maximize your chances of conception and ensure normal, healthy sperm and eggs, it will help to protect the foetus from the risk of abnormalities during the first crucial few weeks after conception.

IMPROVING FERTILITY

Most couples take about six months to conceive, though longer is not unusual. Studies indicate that, if a couple has difficulty conceiving, the man is just as likely to have a fertility problem as the woman. So the health of both partners is very important. Healthy sperm and eggs (ova) are needed to reduce the risk of foetal abnormalities that may lead to miscarriage. Women who smoke are more likely to be infertile, to take longer to conceive, to miscarry and to bleed during pregnancy. If both partners smoke, there is a greater risk of the baby having a low birth weight. Women who drink and smoke are four times more likely to miscarry. Alcohol damages sperm, affects fertility and increases the risk of miscarriage and birth defects. Its effects are greatest in early pregnancy when cell division is at its peak. It is advisable not to drink alcohol from before you hope to conceive until after the birth. If you discover that you are pregnant having not stopped smoking nor reduced your alcohol consumption, do so as soon as possible. Tea and coffee deplete the body of water and valuable minerals, and they are best avoided or strictly limited, along with other drinks containing caffeine.

AVOIDING POLLUTION

Protect yourself from environmental pollution by following these guidelines whenever possible.

- Eat organic, natural and unprocessed foods; wash all fruit.
- Avoid using copper and aluminium cookware.
- Drink filtered or bottled water, not from the tap.
- Avoid heavy traffic and close car windows in tunnels.
- Avoid chemical cleaning agents and pesticides.
- Spend plenty of time outdoors, where sunlight helps to eliminate toxic substances and metabolize benefical minerals.

VITAL NUTRIENTS FOR WOMEN & MEN

NUTRIENT	WOMEN	MEN	DEFICIENCIES
VITAMIN A	*Egg production and reproductive health*	*Healthy sperm*	*Colds, infections, poor skin and hair condition*
B VITAMINS	*Prevents neural tube defects in foetus*	*Male hormone production*	*Irritability, aches and pains, anxiety*
VITAMIN C	*Builds up immunity, body detoxification*	*Improves sperm count and quality*	*Colds, infections, lack of energy*
Zinc	*Egg production and reproductive health*	*Improves sperm count and quality*	*Poor skin condition, poor taste and smell*
OTHER MINERALS	*Reproductive health (magnesium), body detoxification (selenium), balances blood sugar levels (chromium)*	*Improving sperm count (magnesium) and motility (potassium), fertility (selenium)*	*Muscle weakness (magnesium), mental dullness (potassium), nutritional disorders (selenium)*
AMINO ACIDS	*Building and repairing cells and tissues*	*Sperm health and sperm count*	*Muscle weakness, poor wound healing*

EFFECTS OF TOXIC METALS

Each year every person in the industrialized world consumes about 5 kg (11 lb) of additives, absorbs 1 g of heavy metals and has at least 4.5 litres (1 gal) of pesticides or herbicides sprayed on their fruit and vegetables. This toxic overload affects both health and fertility.

• High levels of lead can damage sperm and eggs and affect sperm count and motility. Lead accumulates if calcium, zinc, manganese and iron levels are low. Vitamin C helps to remove lead from the body.

• Mercury from pesticides and fungicides, industrial processes and dental fillings causes loss of libido and impotence.

• Aluminium, for example from saucepans, antiperspirants, food additives and foil-wrapped foods, causes longterm mineral loss and destroys vitamins.

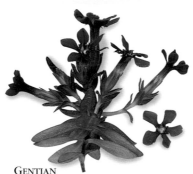

GENTIAN
This flower remedy may help to lift despondency that arises from a difficulty in conceiving.

COMPLEMENTARY THERAPIES

A number of remedies may improve health and fertility.

• Acupuncture (*see pages 134–5*) can help to regulate the menstrual cycle and correct imbalances in body systems. The Chinese believe that a person's every movement, thought, metabolic reaction and sensation is affected by *qi* (life energy), with which we

are endowed from our parents at the moment of conception.

• Flower remedies may also be helpful (*see page 154*). Alpine lily encourages a positive attitude to conception and pregnancy, while bleeding heart may help relieve the grief associated with a previous miscarriage that might prevent conception. Tiger lily may help older women to conceive.

• Osteopathy and chiropractic (*see pages 146–7*) can help to realign the body and restore balance and harmony throughout so that all body parts function as they should.

• Shiatsu (*see page 138*) is believed to improve the body's flow of vital energy, preparing body, mind and spirit for conception and pregnancy.

• Aromatherapy and massage (*see pages 152–3*) can ease stress and relieve physical tension.

Nutrition: Overall Plan

MOTHER AND BABY HAVE DIFFERENT nutritional needs at each stage of pregnancy. Ideally, you should be in peak health before becoming pregnant, so that from the moment of conception your baby has the best chance of development. A good diet throughout pregnancy will ensure your baby's optimum progress.

KEY TIPS

Make sure your diet is balanced, especially if you are vegetarian

*

Eat lots of small meals rather than one or two large ones

*

Avoid highly processed foods, alcohol, tobacco and caffeine

WINDOWS OF OPPORTUNITY

Research shows that while in the womb and immediately after birth, a baby's organs undergo rapid growth spurts. They develop at specific times, in a specific sequence, and for each one there is a specific window of opportunity. These growth spurts affect your baby's health and ability to avoid disease later in life. What you eat may help to maximize these opportunities. The growth of your baby's cells, tissues and organs depends upon an adequate supply of oxygen and essential nutrients. If there are shortages of these, your baby will adapt by slowing cell growth. This slow-down will be especially marked in tissues or organs that are undergoing a critical period of growth. Your health and nutritional status, at the moment of conception and throughout the pregnancy, is of crucial importance to the health and growth of your offspring.

ENERGY REQUIREMENTS

Your body becomes more energy-efficient in pregnancy, increasing your metabolic rate. This affects your need for calories. A pregnant woman's energy requirement is about 1,940 calories a day, increasing by only 200 calories in the third trimester. Appetite is the best indicator of how much to eat. Little and often is the key: five or six small but nutrient-dense meals a day are better than one or two large ones.

RATIONALIZING WEIGHT

Excessive weight gain during pregnancy concerns many women. In general, antenatal clinics no longer weigh women at every visit, it being of limited usefulness. You can weigh yourself at home, of course, remembering to use the same scales, weigh yourself at the same time of day and wear similar clothing each time. The range of weight gain during pregnancy varies, but as a

KEY FOOD TYPES

PROTEINS
These consist of amino acids – the basic building blocks of cells. Foods include meat, fish, cheese, eggs.

CARBOHYDRATES
The main sources of energy, these are simple, such as sugar, or complex, such as starch (pasta, rice, potatoes).

FATS
These are concentrated sources of energy. Some are vital for health, such as polyunsaturated fats, while others (saturated fats) may cause health problems.

VEGETARIAN PASTA
The orange and red peppers, tomatoes and cashews in this vegetarian pasta dish provide rich sources of beta carotene and vitamins C and E.

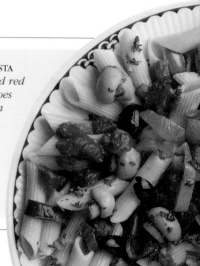

rule you can expect to gain 11–16 kg (24–35 lb): usually 3–4 kg (6–9 lb) in the first 20 weeks and then about 450 g (1 lb) a week thereafter until term. If you are underweight, your gain will be 12.5–18 kg (28–40 lb), and if you are overweight, 7–11 kg (15–25 lb).

VEGETARIAN DIET

A well-balanced vegetarian diet can be nutritionally excellent. Protein from combinations of vegetable sources, such as nuts, pulses and seeds, can be just as good as protein from meat, with the added advantage that they are full of complex carbohydrates and fibre rather than saturated fat. However, pregnant vegetarians must guard against deficiencies, particularly in vitamins B^2, B^6 and B^{12}, zinc, iron and – in the case of vegans – calcium.

MAXIMIZING ABSORPTION

It is important to understand how best to maximize the nutritional value of food.
• Eat organic food preferably and avoid processed and refined foods which contain additives and preservatives.
• Eat food when it is as fresh as possible. Cook vegetables as little as possible (but meat and eggs should be well cooked). Steam food rather than boil it and avoid frying.
• Drink filtered rather than tap water and remember to wash all fruit and vegetables.
• Nutrients work together in synergy, so it is better to take a good multivitamin and mineral supplement than individual minerals or vitamins. Always check that they are suitable for taking during pregnancy. Vitamin A supplements are no longer recommended for pregnant women.
• Eat a wide variety of foods and different coloured foods to include all essential nutrients. To the Chinese, a well-balanced diet means eating the five flavours of foods (sweet, sour, pungent, salty and spicy).

ANTI-NUTRIENTS

Certain substances inhibit the absorption of nutrients.
• The only safe level of alcohol consumption during pregnancy is no alcohol. It

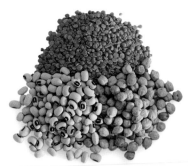

BEANS, CHICKPEAS & LENTILS
A selection of different plant sources of protein eaten every day will supply the amino acids that the body needs.

affects the body's absorption of B vitamins, calcium, iron, zinc and magnesium, and is a factor in raised blood pressure. It can cross the placenta, so if you have a drink, the baby does too.
• Smoking in pregnancy is associated with miscarriage, low birth weight and premature labour. It reduces the supply of oxygen and nutrients to the baby, reducing its growth rate and possibly damaging DNA. Nicotine increases excretion of calcium and destroys vitamin C.
• Tea and coffee have a diuretic effect and interfere with the absorption of calcium, magnesium, zinc and iron.

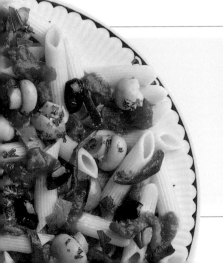

KEY NUTRIENTS NEEDED & SOURCES

CALCIUM
Milk, cheese, yogurt, pulses, nuts, tofu, wholegrains

IRON
Meat, poultry, dark oily fish, pulses, seafood, fortified grains, nuts, seeds, dried fruit, green leafy vegetables

ZINC
Meat, poultry, oysters and other shellfish, pulses, kiwi fruit

B VITAMINS (INCLUDING FOLATE)
Meat, poultry, fish, dairy products, fortified cerals, nuts, seeds, green vegetables, pulses, orange juice, bananas, avocado, wholegrains

VITAMIN C
Citrus fruits, tomatoes, red peppers, strawberries, kiwi fruit, parsley

Boosting Immunity

YOUR NATURAL IMMUNITY is slightly lowered during early pregnancy so that your body does not reject the developing baby. This is part of the normal physiological process of maintaining a pregnancy. With the increasing resistance of bacteria to antibiotics, it is important to maintain a healthy immune system.

KEY TIPS

Reduce stress levels
✻
Eat a healthy, balanced diet
✻
Avoid sources of environmental pollution
✻
Get plenty of sleep

HOW THE IMMUNE SYSTEM WORKS

Disease-producing organisms are to be found in air, food and water and on surfaces that we touch. The immune system defends the body in a number of ways. The first lines of defence are physical barriers – skin and mucous membranes. Mucus is produced by cells in the membranes and this traps bacteria or particles that have been inhaled by the respiratory tract, for example. Buying over-the-counter drugs to dry up a runny nose is not a good idea since it only prolongs this stage of the infection. If a pathogen invades the body successfully, it starts to penetrate cells and proliferate. Chemicals such as histamine in cells alert the immune system to the invader. The blood supply to that area is then increased, moving specialized white blood cells in to attack the invaders.

EFFECTS OF A WEAK SYSTEM

If your immune system is weak you are likely to suffer from recurrent coughs and colds, wounds that are slow to heal, greater fatigue than usual and bacterial, viral or fungal infections. Bacterial infections affect mucous membranes and may be accompanied by fever and swollen lymph glands. Common bacterial infections include boils and impetigo. Viruses invade cells where they replicate. Colds, influenza, warts, herpes and gastroenteritis are all viral infections. Common fungal infections include ringworm and athlete's foot.

CAUSES OF A WEAK SYSTEM

There are several factors that might inhibit or damage your natural immunity.
• Stress and anxiety depresses the immune system.
• Inadequate rest (less than eight hours' sleep a night) can debilitate the immune system.
• Food allergies exhaust the system's defences.
• Diet affects the immune system. Consuming just 80 g (3 oz) of sugar results in a 50 per cent reduction in the activity of white blood cells for between one and five hours. Poor diet generally deprives the body of the nutrients it needs

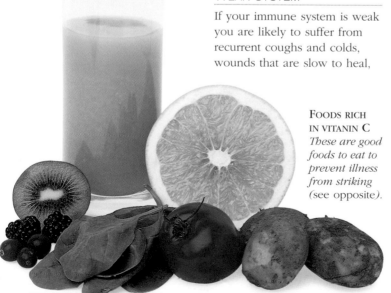

FOODS RICH IN VITANIN C *These are good foods to eat to prevent illness from striking (see opposite).*

EATING FOR HEALTH

NUTRIENT	PROTECTIVE ROLE	FOOD SOURCES
Vitamin A	*Strengthens tissues, cells and mucous membranes*	*Fish oils, egg yolks, cheese, yogurt, carrots, spinach, broccoli, tomatoes*
Vitamin C	*Fights infections, increases resistance to toxins and viruses*	*Most fruit, especially citrus and berries, potatoes, parsley*
Vitamin E	*Protects against free radicals and infections*	*Fresh nuts, seeds, cold-pressed oils*
Zinc	*Fights infections, maintains healthy immune system*	*Ginger, sunflower seeds, cold-pressed oils*
Selenium	*Enhances immune system, fights infection; anti-oxidant*	*Tuna, herring, wheatgerm, Brazil nuts, seafood, seeds*
Green foods	*Enhances immune system, protects against bacteria and viruses*	*Vegetables containing chlorophyll, the green pigment in plants*

for a healthy immune system.
• Alcohol reduces mobilization of white blood cells.
• Air pollution damages mucous membranes.
• Chronic antibiotic use causes general immune impairment.

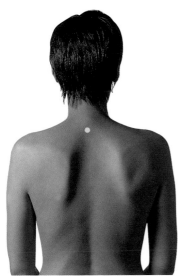

BOOSTING THE IMMUNE SYSTEM
Pressure applied to GV 14 on the back of the neck helps to increase the number of white blood cells.

USING COMPLEMENTARY THERAPIES

Good nutrition is the best foundation on which to build a healthy immune system (*see above*) There are a number of natural ways of boosting the body's immunity.
• **Acupuncture** The Chinese believe that protective *qi* surrounds the body, warding off disease. If the immune system is weak, infection may enter the body, but climatic factors such as wind, cold, heat and damp also play a role. If illness is caused by cold, then an acupuncture point may be warmed. If heat is the cause, certain acupuncture points will be used to clear heat. This therapy can be used to boost the white cell count (*see left*).
• **Aromatherapy** Tea tree oil is an effective antibacterial agent and can be applied topically to fight infection. Inhaling the vapours rising from a few drops of essential oil in hot

water may relieve respiratory infection. Anti-inflammatory oils such as chamomile, lavender, rose and sandalwood will ease bad throats or chest complaints. Breathing difficulties can be eased by using eucalyptus, mint, frankincense or tea tree oils.
• **Herbal remedies** Echinacea is a good, all-round antiviral and antibacterial herb. It can be taken continuously, as capsules or drops, throughout a period of illness, and is perfectly safe during pregnancy. Garlic contains allicin, which has antiviral, antifungal and antibacterial properties. Many regular garlic eaters have been shown to have a lower incidence of cancer. Lemon balm is good for the feverish conditions associated with viral infections, and ginger root, combined with ground cinnamon and lemon and honey to taste, makes a soothing, protective infusion for sore throats and stomach upsets.

Illness during Pregnancy

ILLNESS AND INFECTION ARE NOT KEPT AT BAY just because you have a pregnancy to maintain. The best way of preventing illness is to boost your immune system so that it can fight infection. There are safe and natural remedies that boost immunity and relieve symptoms of some common ailments that strike in pregnancy.

KEY TIPS

Fortify the immune system

✳

Avoid people with infections

✳

Rest, sleep and drink lots of fluids

✳

Consult a doctor if vomiting or diarrhoea persists

COLDS & INFLUENZA

Colds and influenza can be debilitating during pregnancy. Herbal remedies include a warming apple drink made by simmering 15 ml (1 tbsp) concentrated apple juice with 300 ml (½ pint) filtered water, 2.5 g (½ tsp) grated raw ginger, one stick cinnamon and two cloves for 15 minutes, then strain. Drink three cups a day. An infusion (*see page 150*) of elderflower, peppermint or dried yarrow may ease cold symptoms. There are many homeopathic remedies for colds.
• At the first symptoms that develop after being chilled and include a headache, *Aconite 6c*.
• Sudden onset of symptoms, fever, headache, *Belladonna 6c*.
• Aching muscles, joint pain, fever, exhaustion, *Rhus tox 6c*.
• Stuffy nose, watering eyes, headache, sore throat, better for warmth, *Nux vomica 6c*.

PARASITES

Head lice seem to be immune to medicated shampoos and have reached epidemic level among schoolchildren. If you are pregnant, avoid shampoos containing pesticides. Natural solutions include:
• Using a "nit" comb while conditioner is on the hair.
• Adding ten drops geranium or lavender oil to fractionated coconut oil (proportions half and half). Rub into the scalp and leave for one hour before washing off with shampoo.
• Applying diluted tea tree oil (with water, proportions half and half) to the scalp.

CYTOMEGALOVIRUS

Caused by a type of herpes virus, this is common during pregnancy and produces mild influenza-type symptoms. More than half of pregnant women are immune and only a small proportion of those who are not will pass the infection on to the baby, which can cause serious problems. A blood test will reveal immunity status.

CHICKEN POX

This is rare in pregnancy (one in 2,000) since most women have immunity from childhood. A blood test will reveal your immunity status. The virus is

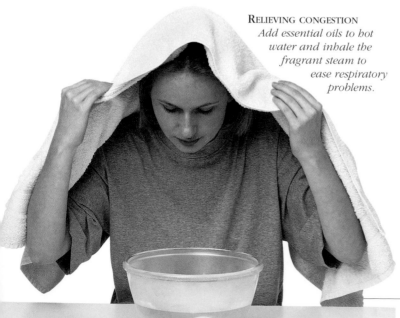

RELIEVING CONGESTION
Add essential oils to hot water and inhale the fragrant steam to ease respiratory problems.

HOMEOPATHIC REMEDIES FOR FOOD INFECTIONS

SYMPTOMS	HOMEOPATHIC REMEDY AND DOSAGE
Burning stomach pains, chilliness, anxiety, thirst, symptoms worse between midnight and 2.00 am	*Arsen. alb. 6c,* every hour for up to 10 doses
Diarrhoea, tearfulness, symptoms worse at night	*Pulsatilla 6c,* every hour for up to 10 doses
Frequent vomiting, bloating, yellow stools, chilliness, symptoms worse for eating	*China 6c,* every hour for up to 10 doses
Diarrhoea worse for movement, rumbling stomach, profuse and watery pale-coloured stools	*Phos. ac. 6c,* every hour for up to 10 doses
Burning stomach pains, blood-streaked stools, violent vomiting, craving for iced water, icy-cold extremities	*Phos. 6c,* every hour for up to 10 doses
Suspected salmonella: painless diarrhoea and fever	*Baptisia 6c,* every hour for up to 10 doses
Unremitting vomiting, foul-smelling greenish-coloured stools	*Ipecac. 6c,* every hour for up to 10 doses

spread by coughs and sneezes and is highly infectious. In the first trimester, especially weeks 1–8, it may cause birth defects, but beyond 12 weeks there is little serious risk until late pregnancy, when you should consult a doctor. Homeopathic remedies can bring relief.

• As a preventative measure if you have been in contact with chicken pox or shingles, *Rhus tox 30c* once a day for ten days.

• At onset of illness, with low fever and general discomfort, *Aconite 30c*; with fever and inflamed spots, *Belladonna 30c*.

• Unbearable itching, *Sulphur 6c*. Rub honey on to the spots, or add ten drops bergamot oil to 5 ml (1 tsp) carrier oil and dab on the spots. Five drops chamomile added to a carrier oil will soothe and heal damaged skin. Use diluted echinacea tincture (with water, half and half) to soothe itching.

FOOD INFECTIONS

Food infections are rare but it is worth avoiding certain foods in pregnancy. These include unpasteurised cheese, especially soft cheeses such as Camembert; blue veined cheeses, such as Danish blue; cook-chill foods; pâté; uncooked eggs, as in homemade ice cream and mayonnaise; and undercooked meat. Always wash fruit and vegetables thoroughly.

• Listeriosis results from eating contaminated soft cheese or chicken. The bacteria crosses the placenta. Infection in the first trimester often results in spontaneous abortion and in the second, premature labour. Infection is rare (1 in 20,000), but the bacterium can survive in temperatures as low as 4°C (39°F) – the typical temperature in a refrigerator.

• Toxoplasmosis is serious during pregnancy. Parasitic in origin, it is contracted by eating or handling raw or undercooked meat or by touching infected cat faeces. The infection can cross the placenta and the greatest risk to the baby is from 10–24 weeks. Spontaneous abortion may occur in early pregnancy and miscarriage and still birth later on. Treatment of toxoplasmosis in pregnancy is complicated as the drugs used can also affect the foetus.

• Salmonella is a common cause of food poisoning (there are 200 different strains). It does not cross the placenta, however. There are a number of homeopathic remedies to treat food infections (*see above*). Herbal remedies include infusions of aniseed, fennel, chamomile or mint, and root ginger (a 2.5 cm /1 in length) added to hot water with a cinnamon stick, lemon juice and honey to taste.

Exercise: Overall Plan

THERE ARE MANY BENEFITS to adopting a regular exercise programme during pregnancy. Exercise will boost energy levels, maintain and promote circulation and mobility, and encourage good posture by increasing physical awareness and control. Exercise can also target certain muscles in preparation for labour.

PHYSIOLOGICAL CHANGES

Changes in pregnancy affect every body system and must be taken into account before exercising. Hormonal changes are highly significant. Relaxin, produced from two weeks into pregnancy and reaching a peak at 12 weeks, relaxes ligaments so that the pelvis can expand during delivery. Ligaments throughout the body are also relaxed, however, and the stability of joints is affected. It is easy to overstretch, putting the spine and pelvis at risk. Progesterone modifies the diaphragm and the ribs flare slightly to allow more room for the growing uterus. An increase in girth and weight means that your posture will change and your centre of gravity will shift. You may find it hard to co-ordinate movements and to balance. The amount of blood pumped by the heart increases by up to 40 per cent during pregnancy and the size of the heart increases to cope with this.

GENERAL GUIDELINES

Pregnancy is not the time to start aerobics classes unless they are especially structured for pregnancy. If you are used to doing such exercise and do not want to let your fitness level drop, continue but bear in mind the following guidelines.
• Your heart rate should not rise above 140 beats a minute. Do not do strenuous exercise for more than 15 minutes.

• Several research studies have indicated that intensive exercise raises the mother's core body temperature and causes vasoconstriction (the narrowing of blood vessels), which reduces blood flow and hence oxygen supply to the uterus, with a corresponding rise in the foetal heart rate.
• Increased body mass creates momentum that makes it more difficult to control movements. Jerky movements, bouncing and jumping should be avoided because impact is transmitted to the joints. Whatever stage of pregnancy you are at, be guided by your body.
• Never force yourself to exercise beyond what feels comfortable. Avoid unstable positions, such as standing on one leg for a long time. In each trimester consider the most appropriate exercise (*see pages 32–3, 50–1* and *74–5*). Always warm up before doing any exercise and cool down when you have finished (*see page 32*).

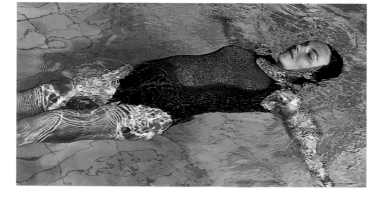

AQUAROBICS
Exercising in water is beneficial because there is less stress on the joints and on uterine blood flow.

CHOOSING EXERCISE

Seek out specially structured pregnancy fitness classes, which have a cardiovascular section, a muscle-strengthening section and a cool-down. Any strenuous exercise should be limited to 15 minutes and you should always be supervised by a teacher who is aware of the physiological changes that take place during pregnancy. Apart from exercise classes, gentle cycling is good exercise in pregnancy, although your changing centre of gravity may be a problem latterly. Walking is excellent, and speed walking is preferable to running or jogging. Swimming and water-based exercise are ideal forms of exercise. The resistance of the water enhances the effects of exercise, and strain on the back is relieved while the uterus is supported by the water. Contact sports such as hockey or netball should be avoided.

SEASONAL EXERCISE

The idea of living one's life in harmony with nature is fundamental to Traditional Chinese Medicine. In the five element theory, the seasons of the year and the changes that they bring affect our growth and well-being (*see pages 133*). The Chinese believe that exercise – as well as diet and lifestyle habits – need to be adjusted according to these seasonal changes (*see below*).

EXERCISE IN HARMONY WITH NATURE

THE CHINESE BELIEVE THAT, *pregnant or not, you should adjust your exercise regime to suit the time of year in order to be in harmony with your surroundings. Different seasons lend themselves to different exercises. Spring, summer and late summer are the* yang *seasons, while autumn and winter are* yin *seasons. If preconceptual care is included, a pregnancy lasts in effect for 12 months and all five seasons.*

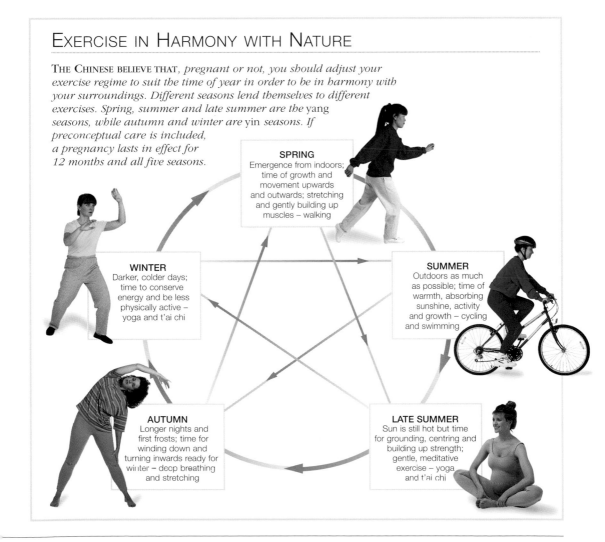

SPRING
Emergence from indoors; time of growth and movement upwards and outwards; stretching and gently building up muscles – walking

WINTER
Darker, colder days; time to conserve energy and be less physically active – yoga and t'ai chi

SUMMER
Outdoors as much as possible; time of warmth, absorbing sunshine, activity and growth – cycling and swimming

AUTUMN
Longer nights and first frosts; time for winding down and turning inwards ready for winter – deep breathing and stretching

LATE SUMMER
Sun is still hot but time for grounding, centring and building up strength; gentle, meditative exercise – yoga and t'ai chi

At Home & at Work

WHETHER AT HOME OR AT WORK, your surroundings exert influence over your stress levels, state of health and general well-being. Organize the places in which you spend most of your time, harnessing your natural "nesting" instincts to create harmony, positive energy and a pleasant, calm-inducing atmosphere.

CHINESE BELIEFS

Feng shui is the Chinese art of understanding and harnessing the universal flow of *qi* energy around the home and in places of work. It is believed that this energy can be a positive force in life, for happiness, prosperity and good health. Feng shui includes a number of ideas to enhance your home. There are other, simple, common-sense measures that will help to improve your surroundings.

• Use mirrors and reflective surfaces to capture pleasant views from outside and, the Chinese believe, reflect bad energy out of a building.

• Wind chimes and bells can help to break up stagnant *qi*, but are not advisable in a bedroom.

• Fresh flowers and plants bring good *yang* energy into a building, but make sure you replace dead ones. Some people believe that you should not have plants in a bedroom, but that fruits are an excellent idea. The pomegranate, in particular, is associated with fertility symbolism.

• Air all rooms and replace stale energy once a day by opening the windows and encouraging a through draught.

• Decorating a bedroom in red is said to stimulate passion and to bring good luck to couples wishing to start a family. You may, however, prefer a colour scheme for your bedroom that is associated more with relaxation, such as pale green.

• Make sure your mattress is comfortable and gives your body the correct support.

• Have your windows double-glazed, or hang heavy curtains if the room is noisy.

• Tidy away books, newspapers and discarded clothes to help create the impression of your bedroom being a sanctuary and a haven of tranquillity.

IMPROVING YOUR SURROUNDINGS
Fresh flowers, scented candles, incense, essential oils and crystals improve a room's atmosphere.

CLEARING SPACE

As you prepare to welcome a new human being into your life, find time to sort out your home and dispose of unwanted things and clutter. This will help to create space for your new baby, both literally and psychologically. If you are decorating, imagine introducing light, happiness and harmony as you choose colours and fabrics. Bring fresh flowers into your home, light candles and incense, or spray the rooms with water containing a few drops of essential oil of lavender, mandarin or grapefruit.

AVOIDING POLLUTION

To minimalize the risks from the environment, bear in mind the following general precautions.
• Avoid standing immediately in front of a microwave oven while it is in use.
• Avoid living close to high-voltage cables during pregnancy.
• Avoid chemical hazards such as oven cleaners, garden pesticides and chemical-based cleaning agents. Check the contents of products you are using, and opt for safe, natural alternatives whenever possible.
• Avoid driving in heavy traffic and always close car windows when passing through tunnels.
• Wash all fruit and vegetables and remove the outer leaves of vegetables. Eat organic produce whenever possible.
• Avoid using aluminium or copper cookware and do not wrap food in aluminium foil.

COPING WITH WORK

Unless your work is physically demanding or the work environment is hazardous, there is no reason why you should not work through pregnancy until about 32 weeks. You may need to make some adjustments to your working day, however.
• If you spend long periods of time in front of a VDU, make sure that you sit with the screen at the correct distance and height, and that you take short, frequent breaks away from it.
• Make your day less arduous by sitting down as much as possible, putting your feet up and resting if at all possible (*see below*). Do not be afraid to ask for help if you need it and take a break if you feel fatigued.
• Make sure that you know the details of your maternity entitlements as well as your obligations to your employer.

USING COMPLEMENTARY THERAPIES

There are several gentle ways of nurturing more positive, stress-free surroundings.
• The flower remedy yarrow special formula may be of benefit if you are exposed to environmental stresses during pregnancy, including radiation or any form of toxicity. It is especially useful if you have to travel during pregnancy, particularly by air. (You should avoid flying during the first trimester, especially if you have a history of miscarriage.) This remedy can be taken internally but also applied topically to the abdomen.
• Quartz crystals may be of benefit around the home and workplace. Place crystals near your computer, for example, if you spend a great deal of time in front of it. Amber crystals, citrine and tourmaline are believed by some to offer a degree of protection from electromagnetic fields and radiation. Hanging a bright crystal above the entrance to your home is thought to encourage *qi* into the building.

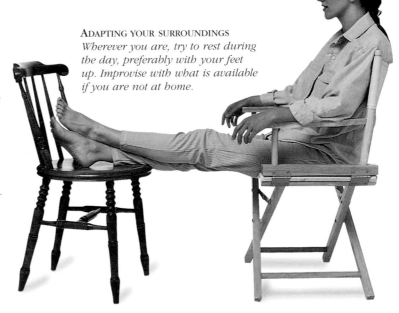

ADAPTING YOUR SURROUNDINGS
Wherever you are, try to rest during the day, preferably with your feet up. Improvise with what is available if you are not at home.

Antenatal Checks

ALL PREGNANT WOMEN ARE MONITORED routinely throughout their pregnancy at antenatal visits to a midwife or doctor. A range of tests may be recommended in order to detect foetal abnormalities, depending on the mother's medical or family history, experience in previous pregnancies, or her age.

KEY TIPS

Carry your maternity notes with you

＊

Take time to consider carefully any special antenatal tests that you are offered

＊

Do not miss an antenatal visit

ROUTINE TESTS

At your first antenatal visit, a midwife will take your medical history and advise you about diet, smoking and drinking alcohol. She will take a blood sample and feel your abdomen. At this and subsequent visits, your blood pressure will be checked and urine tested. It depends on your hospital, but appointments are usually every four weeks until week 28, then every two weeks until week 36, and then weekly. All working women are entitled to be paid during antenatal visits.

BLOOD & URINE TESTS

Blood tests check blood group, haemoglobin levels (to see if you are anaemic) and immunity to rubella (if you are not

FOETAL HEARTBEAT
Listening to the foetal heartbeat for the first time can be very reassuring and reinforces the bond with your baby.

immune you will be offered a postnatal vaccination). They also test for syphilis, diabetes, hepatitis and your rhesus status. A rhesus negative mother with a rhesus positive baby will be given "anti-D" immunization at 28 weeks and after the birth. Rhesus disease may otherwise affect subsequent rhesus-positive children as the mother produces anti-rhesus positive antibodies. The blood-pressure reading taken at your first antenatal visit will be the one that every subsequent reading is measured against, so try to be as relaxed as possible. It is normal for your blood pressure to rise a little in late pregnancy. Urine is checked for ketones (which reduce the efficiency of oxygen transportation in the

ANTENATAL CHECKS

TRANSVAGINAL SCAN Carried out from 5–6 weeks. A probe is inserted into the vagina giving a clear view of the growing baby.	ADVANTAGES *results are instant.* DISADVANTAGES *baby exposed to high-frequency sound.*
CVS (CHORIONIC VILLUS SAMPLING) Detects chromosomal and genetic disorders such as Down's syndrome and sickle-cell anaemia. A tube is inserted into the uterus at 8–12 weeks and cells taken from placental tissue surrounding the embryo.	ADVANTAGES *very accurate and preliminary results within 48 hours.* DISADVANTAGES *risk of miscarriage (roughly one in 100).*
NUCHAL TEST Non-invasive ultrasound scan carried out at 12 weeks to detect chromosomal disorders. "Nuchal" means neck: the scan checks for abnormal thickness in the fold at the back of the baby's neck. When combined with a blood test, the nuchal test is 80–90 per cent in accurate in predicting Down's syndrome.	ADVANTAGES *non invasive and no risk of miscarriage.* DISADVANTAGES *none.*
AFP (ALPHA-FETOPROTEIN TEST) Blood test that checks blood protein levels and detects neurological problems such as spina bifida or hydrocephalus. Carried out at 15–18 weeks. Accuracy is not good: high and low levels of alpha-fetoprotein can be found in women carrying perfectly normal babies and those who are very nauseous. Results take about 10 days.	ADVANTAGES *non-invasive with no side effects.* DISADVANTAGES *only 50 per cent accurate; false-positive rate of 5–10 per cent.*
AMNIOCENTESIS Sample of amniotic fluid taken under local anaesthetic through the abdominal wall at 16–18 weeks. Cells are tested for many disorders, including Down's syndrome. Results in 2–3 weeks.	ADVANTAGES *very accurate (about 90 per cent); reveals baby's sex (important with some disorders).* DISADVANTAGES *risk of miscarriage (less than one in 100); discomfort; possible side effects (bleeding, infection); screens few defects.*
TRIPLE/QUADRUPLE/LEEDS/BART'S TESTS Combination of blood tests to assess risk of chromosomal defects or problems such as anencephaly (absence of a brain) or spina bifida.	ADVANTAGES *no risk of miscarriage.* DISADVANTAGES *accuracy between 60 and 80 per cent.*

blood), protein (which might indicate pre-eclampsia or an infection) and sugar. A glucose tolerance test (GTT) may be necessary to check for diabetes.

ULTRASOUND SCANNING

This is routine at 16–18 weeks. High-pitched sound waves are reflected back off the baby and reproduced electronically on a screen as an image. It confirms dates and multiple pregnancies, detects certain abnormalities and checks the position of the placenta. A scan is painless and there is no risk of miscarriage.

SPECIAL TESTS

You need to think long and hard about special antenatal tests (*see above*). Most of them are not obligatory. Make sure that you understand exactly what you are being offered and why, and if there will be any risk to your baby. Explore any alternatives before making a decision. You should consider that often your only option, should the results of any tests be positive, will be whether or not to terminate the pregnancy. Support and counselling will be on hand, however, in case of such an eventuality.

Out-of-the-ordinary Pregnancies

CERTAIN KINDS OF PREGNANCY are believed to put the foetus at a higher risk than normal. If you have any complications whatsoever, you will be monitored closely by medical professionals throughout your pregnancy. You will need to pay particular attention to your nutrition and other aspects of your lifestyle.

MULTIPLE PREGNANCIES

More women are giving birth to twins or triplets as a result of fertility treatment. A multiple pregnancy is not high-risk as such, but you are unlikely to go to term and, because of the possibility of complications during the birth, you will be advised against a home birth. You are also more likely to experience minor ailments such as morning sickness, heartburn, backache, sleeplessness, fatigue and raised blood pressure (*see pages 36–43, 54–67 and 78–91*). Plenty of rest and a good diet make good foundations for a multiple pregnancy. Great demands are made on your stores of iron and folate, for example, if you are carrying more than one baby so you could easily become anaemic.

OLDER MOTHERS

Many more women are having babies later in life. The older you are, the more important diet and lifestyle become. You will generally be advised to give up work as early as you can, rest as much as you can (particularly between 5 pm and 7 pm – *see page 132*) and eat

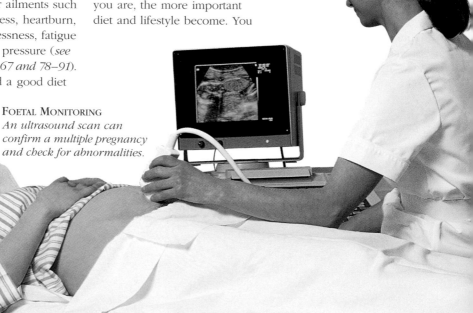

FOETAL MONITORING
An ultrasound scan can confirm a multiple pregnancy and check for abnormalities.

as healthy a diet as you can (*see pages 12–13*). This should include a good vitamin and mineral supplement.

IVF PREGNANCIES

Good preparation for in vitro fertilization (IVF) is essential. Women having this treatment tend to be older and to suffer what the Chinese regard as Kidney deficiency and weak *jing*, both of which can be corrected by acupuncture. Be sure to take time off work and rest completely at the time of egg transfer. Eat a diet rich in zinc and essential fatty acids, important for cell division and healthy cell membranes.

PREMATURE LABOUR

A premature labour is one that starts six weeks or more before your due date. If you went into labour early in a previous pregnancy, the chances are that you will do so again. Acupuncture may help if you have a history of premature birth but you need to start treatment in mid-pregnancy. Plenty of rest and good nutrition are both important. Make sure you have adequate supplies of essential fatty acids and zinc and iron, since deficiencies in these have been linked with premature labour. Watch out for symptoms of a urinary infection, which can cause premature labour, or low backache, which may indicate the start of labour.

DIABETES

Gestational diabetes develops during pregnancy and affects around five per cent of women who previously had no history of diabetes. This potentially serious condition usually develops during the second half of pregnancy and will be detected by routine antenatal urine tests. This condition will make you more prone to infections such as cystitis and thrush and to raised blood pressure. Induction or a Caesarean section may be recommended at 36 weeks. You will be closely monitored by your midwife or obstetrician and a nutritionist. Controlling diabetes by dietary measures requires care and self-discipline: eat little and often, choose your food carefully (*see below*) and limit alcohol consumption. Constitutional homeopathic treatment (*see pages 148–9*), for which you will need to consult a practitioner, may help.

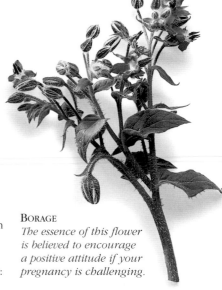

BORAGE
The essence of this flower is believed to encourage a positive attitude if your pregnancy is challenging.

REDUCING SUGAR INTAKE

If you have sugar in your urine, you should avoid certain foods. You can eat as much as you like of others.

FOODS TO AVOID
• Sugar, fizzy drinks, cordials and squashes, biscuits and cakes, sweet puddings and some canned foods
• Fatty foods
• Salt and salty foods
• Highly processed foods

FOODS TO EAT FREELY
• Starchy foods such as bread, pasta, rice, noodles and cereals
• Fruit and vegetables
• Pulses
• Low-fat alternatives

COMPLEMENTARY THERAPIES IN HIGH-RISK PREGNANCIES

If your pregnancy is at all high-risk, it is important that any complementary therapy you consider is taken in conjunction with conventional treatment and advice from your midwife and doctor and in their full knowledge. Consult qualified complementary practitioners and inform them of your condition. Flower remedies are gentle and may be of help to a number of conditions. Angelica is generally beneficial in early pregnancy if you have a history of miscarriage; borage is said to lift the spirits if circumstances surrounding your pregnancy are difficult; California wild rose is generally useful for difficult pregnancies; gentian is good for coping with setbacks during pregnancy; mariposa lily helps to encourage a positive outlook and is useful at all stages of pregnancy; while tiger lily promotes a successful pregnancy in older women.

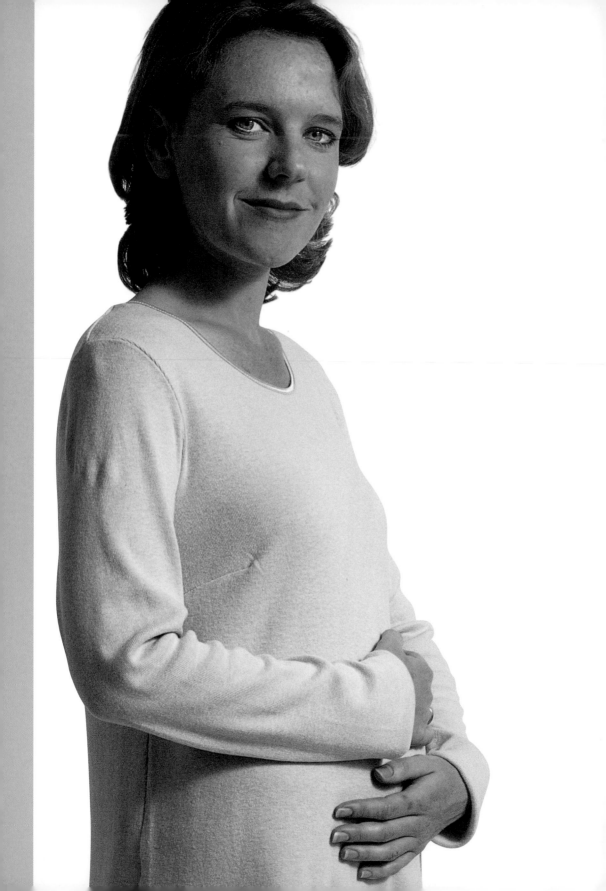

THE FIRST THREE MONTHS OF PREGNANCY are exciting but they can also give rise to anxiety. You and your partner may feel that it is too early to share your news with family and friends, but you are having to come to terms with great changes, not only to your body but also to both your lives. You will need time to adjust to the

The first trimester

idea of parenthood, and with this will come emotional highs and lows. This chapter addresses some of your natural anxieties, offers advice on how to keep as well as possible in terms of diet and exercise, and suggests how to deal with minor ailments that may affect you during this early stage of pregnancy.

Development of Mother & Baby

THE DEVELOPMENT OF A BABY TAKES 38 WEEKS from conception (40 weeks of pregnancy is calculated from the first day of your last menstrual period). By the third week after conception, you may realize that your period is late and suspect that you are pregnant.

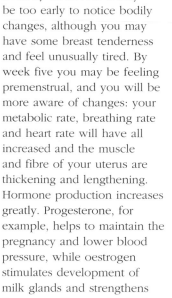

> ### KEY TIPS
>
> *Consider antenatal tests carefully: they are not compulsory*
>
> ✳
>
> *Eat little and often if you are feeling nauseous*
>
> ✳
>
> *Rest if you feel tired*
>
> ✳
>
> *Accept that it may take time to adjust to being pregnant*

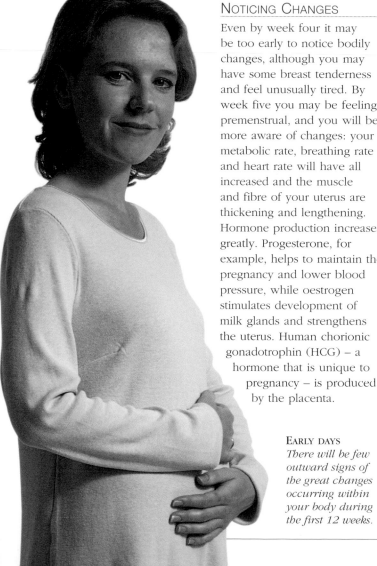

NOTICING CHANGES

Even by week four it may be too early to notice bodily changes, although you may have some breast tenderness and feel unusually tired. By week five you may be feeling premenstrual, and you will be more aware of changes: your metabolic rate, breathing rate and heart rate will have all increased and the muscle and fibre of your uterus are thickening and lengthening. Hormone production increases greatly. Progesterone, for example, helps to maintain the pregnancy and lower blood pressure, while oestrogen stimulates development of milk glands and strengthens the uterus. Human chorionic gonadotrophin (HCG) – a hormone that is unique to pregnancy – is produced by the placenta.

EARLY DAYS
There will be few outward signs of the great changes occurring within your body during the first 12 weeks.

Hormonal changes may cause great emotional highs and lows as well as nausea and sickness.

MAKING PLANS

By week six your pregnancy will have been confirmed. Contact your midwife or doctor and arrange for your first visit to an antenatal clinic between weeks eight and 12. Also make an appointment to see your dentist to maintain healthy teeth and gums. You will be aware of the speeding up of your metabolism. You may feel drained – as if someone has "pulled the plug". By about week eight you may experience mild abdominal pains as your uterus starts to stretch. If you suffer severe abdominal pain, see your doctor immediately. By week nine you should be thinking about antenatal tests. There are several screening and diagnostic tests to detect foetal abnormalities, but consider the implications of a positive result (*see page 23*). By week 12 the uterus is starting to move out of the pelvis, becoming an abdominal organ, and the heart is pumping extra blood.

THE BABY'S DEVELOPMENT

1 WEEK 1 After fertilization, the sperm and ovum nuclei fuse to form a zygote. This starts to divide as it travels to the uterus.

2 WEEK 2 After six or seven days, the cell mass develops a hollow cavity and is now called a blastocyst. By the tenth day it becomes embedded in the endometrium.

3 WEEK 3 The blastocyst is the size of a pinhead but is multiplying fast. The inner cells of the cavity develop into the embryo.

4 WEEK 4 The baby is about 2 mm (¹⁄₁₆ in) in length and weighs less than 1 gm (³⁄₁₀₀ oz). Its body tissues are forming from three embryonic layers: the hair, nails, mammary glands, teeth enamel, inner ear and lenses for the eyes from one layer; the nervous system, retina, pituitary gland, muscle, cartilage, bones, blood and lymph cells from another; and lungs, trachea, liver, pancreas and bladder from a third.

5 WEEK 5 The heart has started to develop: it now has four chambers. The roof palate of the mouth is forming.

6 WEEK 6 The cluster of cells is becoming an embryo, roughly the size of a fingertip. The heart is beating at 180 beats a minute, more than twice as fast as yours. Eyelids, ears, and the beginnings of hands and feet are forming. The shape of the head and the curve of the spine are discernible.

7 WEEK 7 The embryo has quadrupled in size and the nervous system is developing well. The baby is starting to move its body, arms and legs. These movements can be detected by a monitor, but you will not be able to feel them. The lungs, liver and kidneys are starting to develop.

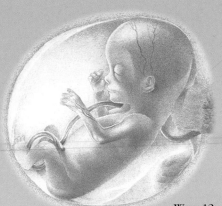

WEEK 12

8 WEEK 8 About 2.5 cm (1 in) in length, the embryo has now evolved into a foetus. Its brain is developing rapidly, and the umbilical cord has formed. Ears are beginning to develop and the mouth is able to open and close.

9 WEEK 9 The baby is now 4 cm (1½ in) in length and can wriggle slightly. The digestive and nervous systems are developing fast and the brain is four times larger than it was four weeks ago.

10 WEEK 10 The nervous system has matured enough for the baby to move about more. All the organs plus the sack of amniotic fluid have been formed and the baby is now recognizable as a human being.

11 WEEK 11 The liver takes over the manufacture of red blood cells and the kidneys are functioning. The baby is about 5 cm (2 in) long and growing rapidly. It has a completely formed face. The head is growing to accommodate the brain.

12 WEEK 12 Your baby is fully formed, although, at just 6 cm (2½ in) long, there is a lot of growing still to do. Its nails and hair are starting to grow, its jaw has 32 little teeth buds, and it is starting to suck. Internal sex organs have formed.

Nutrition for Mother & Baby

THE FIRST THREE MONTHS OF PREGNANCY are in many ways the most crucial for your baby's healthy development. A poor diet may affect the formation of organs and the development of body systems, as well as leading to a reduced birth weight. Certain vitamins and minerals are particularly important.

KEY TIPS

Eat little and often if you are feeling nauseous

✳

Include plenty of iron-rich foods in your diet

✳

Take a folic acid supplement

FUELLING DEVELOPMENT

Nutrition prior to conception is extremely important (*see pages 10–13*). This, in effect, extends into pregnancy, in that many women do not discover that they are pregnant until four or five weeks after conception. By this time many important developments have already occurred in the embryo. By the end of 12 weeks, a baby is fully formed, and the framework for all the organs, limbs, muscles, and bones is already in place (*see pages 29*).

KEY NUTRIENTS

Of the key food types, protein is needed in large amounts by the mother for building and repairing cells, muscles, organs, tissues and hair, and for enzyme production. At least half the calories should come from carbohydrates, mainly in the form of starch. Of the key nutrients needed at this time, folate and iron are vitally important. Folate is a B vitamin used for cell division, red blood cell formation, and development of the baby's nervous system. Since the neural tube forms in the fourth week of gestation, you should boost folate supplies by taking a folic acid supplement before you conceive to help to prevent defects such as spina bifida. Folate levels are difficult to maintain from food alone so you may need to continue the supplement. Iron is found in haemoglobin, and is needed to transport oxygen and carbon dioxide, to make enzymes and to generate energy. The demand for iron increases in pregnancy due to an increase in blood volume in an expectant woman and the development of the placenta.

KEY DAILY DIETARY CONSTITUENTS

6 servings of grains

5 servings of vegetables

2 servings of lean meat, fish or pulses

2 servings of folic-acid-rich foods

2 servings of calcium-rich foods

Plenty of filtered or mineral water

SUMMER VEGETABLES
Roasted red and yellow peppers, tomatoes, cucumber, anchovies and eggs provide a substantial main-course salad dish.

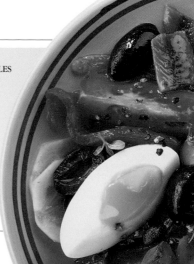

ESSENTIAL DIETARY NUTRIENTS

VITAMINS & MINERALS	FOR MOTHER	FOR BABY
VITAMIN A Some of your intake of beta carotene may be converted into vitamin A.	*For its anti-oxidant properties and to fight infection.*	*For cell differentiation, eye development, formation of healthy cell membranes.*
B VITAMINS You do not need to increase intakes unless you are adolescent, carrying twins or at risk of diabetes.	*B^2 and B^6 to balance hormones; B^2 and B^5 for energy; B^6 to improve metabolism.*	*B^{12} for nervous system; B^6 for healthy immune system and brain development.*
OTHER VITAMINS The need for vitamin D increases in pregnancy, and also for vitamin E if consumption of polyunsaturated fats is high.	*C for iron absorption and hormone production; D to absorb and utilize calcium.*	*D for healthy bones; E for the developing heart.*
FOLATE	*See Key Nutrients, opposite.*	*See Key Nutrients, opposite.*
IRON	*See Key Nutrients, opposite.*	*See Key Nutrients, opposite.*
CALCIUM The foetus accumulates calcium rapidly during the first trimester.	*For healthy bones and teeth.*	*For muscle contraction and nerve transmission.*
ZINC Essential throughout pregnancy.	*For production of hormones.*	*For cell reproduction and growth; to prevent low birth weight.*
OTHER MINERALS Good iodine levels are needed prior to conception. Chromium may prevent nausea. Magnesium may prevent raised blood pressure.	*Manganese and chromium for blood sugar regulation; manganese and magnesium for hormone balance and energy production.*	*Manganese for prevention of foetal malformations; iodine to prevent hyperthyroidism.*

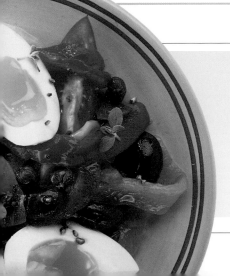

SUGGESTED MEAL PLAN

BREAKFAST
Oatflake cereal with sesame seeds, banana, pear and milk

MIDMORNING SNACK
Apple, oatcake and slice of Cheddar cheese

LUNCH
Mackerel with watercress, grated carrot and tomato; wholemeal bread and butter; an orange

AFTERNOON SNACK
Dried figs and almonds

DINNER
Lamb and black-eyed bean casserole, potatoes, carrots and broccoli

BEDTIME SNACK
Pure fruit blueberry jam with wholemeal bread and butter

Exercise Plan

HUGE EMOTIONAL AND PHYSICAL CHANGES take place during the early months of pregnancy. Some women worry about their level of fitness and want to rush straight into an exercise programme, while others struggle to cope with the emotional roller-coaster and the fatigue typical of early pregnancy.

KEY TIPS

Stop exercising if you experience serious discomfort or pain

✳

Do not over-exert yourself

✳

Do not get overheated

✳

Set yourself realistic targets

WARMING UP & COOLING DOWN

IT IS IMPORTANT *to warm up when you start exercising. The aim of a warm-up is to mobilize major joints – by means of static stretches – then to move the joints to warm them up. This is* *followed by aerobic exercise that raises the pulse further and strengthens the muscles. You should then cool down, stretching out muscles that have been worked. Finally, relax the body.*

GENERAL GUIDELINES

You should at all times be aware of general guidelines relating to exercise during pregnancy (*see pages 18–19*).

MOBILIZING JOINTS

Work through the body, starting from the top.

• **Head and neck** Sitting cross-legged, turn the head slowly and smoothly from side to side 6–8 times. Then, lower the ear towards the shoulder and lift it back up. Repeat 6–8 times on each side. Turn the head to one side and slowly sweep the chin across the chest to the other side. Repeat 6–8 times on each side.

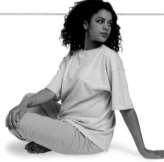

• **Shoulders and arms** Lift the right shoulder and lower, then the left. Repeat 6–8 times. Then, pull both shoulders forward, lift and push back. Do this 6–8 times, then repeat rotating forwards. Finally, kneel and sit on your heels. Stretch the right arm up and bend it so that your hand is behind your back. Use the left hand to push the elbow gently backwards to increase the stretch (*see left*). Repeat with the left arm.

• **Spine and pelvis** Sit with legs crossed, back straight and neck stretched slightly upwards. Breathing out, turn the upper body to the right, placing your right hand behind you for stability (*see centre left*). Put the left hand on the right knee and use it to push your body slightly further round. Repeat to the left. Then, stand with feet hip-width apart, knees soft, and hips and feet facing forwards. Rotate the upper body slowly in each direction several times. Do the same with the hips. Finally, tucking the bottom under and tilting the pelvis upwards, tighten the abdominal muscles.

• **Hips and legs** Stand with feet slightly wider than hip-width apart, knees soft, bottom tucked under and pelvis tilted upwards. Lift the right hip and hold for five seconds. Repeat 6–8 times, then with the left hip. Sitting with legs out and leaning on the arms for support, bend each leg and straighten it several times (*see below*).

WORKING HARDER

Once you have mobilized the joints, combine two or three gentle, low-impact aerobic steps into a five-minute programme to move the joints and warm them up and raise the pulse slightly.

This might include marching backwards and forwards, marching on the spot with knee-lifts, side-steps with half-squats and transfer-of-weight steps such as hamstring curls. Finally in the warm-up, gently stretch out muscles that have been worked to ease tension out of them. Next, proceed to aerobic work to maintain or improve your stamina and cardiovascular function, increase oxygen supply to all parts of the body and improve body awareness. While not raising your fitness level, this part of your exercise programme will equip you to deal with the physical demands of pregnancy and labour. Use the same steps as before, just make them more dynamic, and combine several into a 15-minute programme.

• **Hamstring curls** Step on to the right foot, bending the left leg and bringing the left foot up towards the bottom. Swing your arms from side to side. Repeat, stepping to the left.

MUSCLE STRENGTH & ENDURANCE

Pregnant women should target specific muscles to improve posture and prepare them for labour and life beyond the birth. So, after your aerobic work, do exercises to strengthen the upper body, such as pec-decks and box-position press-ups, to help with bending and lifting, for example. Exercises for the lower body include side leg-lifts or static half-squats on the spot. Other exercises may help to relieve aches and pains (*see below*). Stretch out all muscles used in a final cool-down.

MARCHING
Walking briskly will increase your heart rate, improving cardiovascular function.

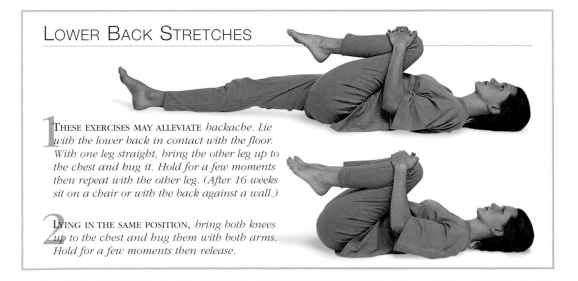

LOWER BACK STRETCHES

1 THESE EXERCISES MAY ALLEVIATE *backache. Lie with the lower back in contact with the floor. With one leg straight, bring the other leg up to the chest and hug it. Hold for a few moments then repeat with the other leg. (After 16 weeks sit on a chair or with the back against a wall.)*

2 LYING IN THE SAME POSITION, *bring both knees up to the chest and hug them with both arms. Hold for a few moments then release.*

Five-point Action Plan

THE FIRST THREE MONTHS of pregnancy are an exciting but possibly also a nerve-wracking time, whether your baby is planned or a surprise. During these first few weeks, you will be coming to terms not only with the physical changes to your body but with the impact that a new baby is going to have on your life. The following advice may be helpful.

GET ENOUGH SLEEP

A good night's sleep is the best foundation on which to start each day. You may find yourself in bed by 8 pm each evening, as you respond to your body's needs. Promote restful sleep by eating a light supper at the end of the day so as not to overload your digestive system before you go to bed. Try and put your feet up during the day and catnap during the afternoon, if work or other children permit.

TAKE TIME TO ADJUST

You will experience emotional highs and lows, and you may feel more exhausted than ever before. You will have many decisions to make: when to tell people your news; when to stop work; what childcare provisions need to be made. Many people prefer to keep their news a secret for the first three months, waiting until they are more confident about their pregnancy. Do not rush decisions: take time to adjust and make plans.

EXERCISE SENSIBLY

Do not force yourself to exercise at this stage of pregnancy if you do not feel like it. Gentle forms of exercise such as walking, stretching and swimming are preferable to a strenuous work-out in the gym. More research is needed on the possible effects of the mother's increased body temperature as a result of exertion on the formation of her baby's vital organs during the first three months. Do not over-exert yourself or get overheated.

IMPROVE YOUR DIET

Take a good look at what you eat. Vitamins and minerals are often eliminated by modern methods of cultivation, food processing and cooking. The chances are that you lack the full complement of nutrients needed while your baby's organs are forming. Try to eat fresh organic food, take a good all-round multivitamin and a folic acid supplement, and avoid alcohol, tea, coffee and highly processed foods.

PREPARE MENTALLY

Take time out each day to be quiet and calm and to reflect upon what is happening to you and how your life is changing. Apart from all the practical considerations that you need to give thought to, it is also important to start to form a relationship with your unborn baby by visualizing the child. Listen to music if it helps to soothe your mind and relax your body.

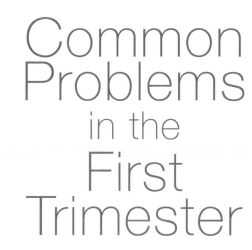

Common Problems in the First Trimester

THIS CAN BE AN ANXIOUS TIME, when you are not yet fully confident about your pregnancy. You may also feel very drained of energy and emotion. The following pages will help you to deal with some of the minor ailments that are common in early pregnancy.

Morning Sickness

ABOUT HALF OF PREGNANT WOMEN experience morning sickness. It is most likely to affect those with nutritional deficiencies. The development of the placenta and associated hormone levels, which peak at 9–10 weeks, may be responsible, but vomiting can also be the body's way of eliminating toxins.

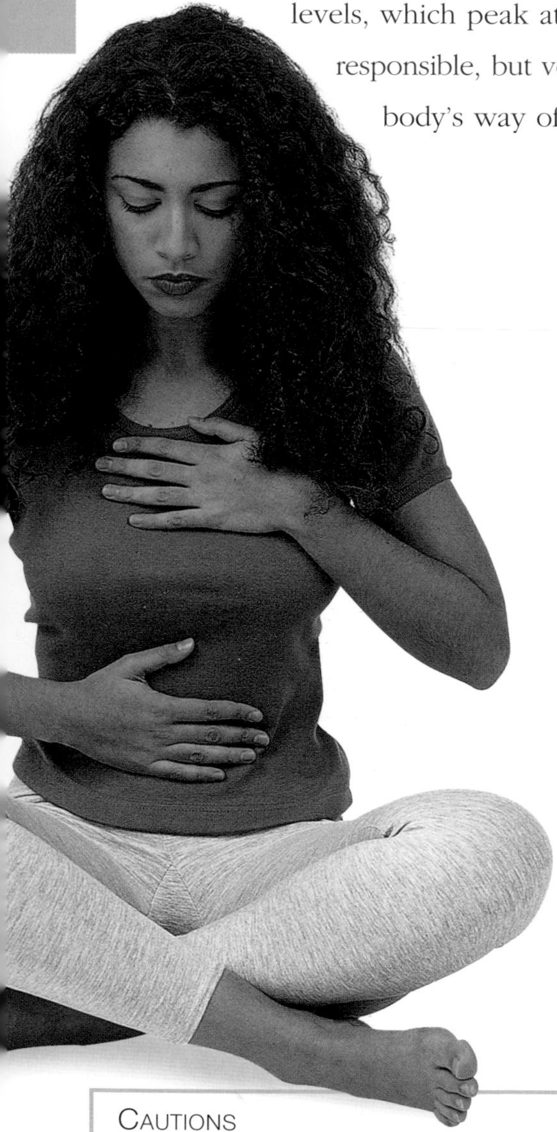

SYMPTOMS

Nausea and vomiting

✳

Excessive salivation

✳

Disinclination to eat

✳

Side effect: fatigue

DIET & NUTRITION

Eat foods that appeal to you and are easy to prepare, and eat frequently as this stabilizes blood sugar levels. Your need for vitamins B^6 and B^{12}, folic acid, iron and zinc increases in pregnancy. Nausea is linked with B^6 and zinc deficiencies in particular. If you vomit a lot you may also develop a magnesium deficiency. Vitamin and mineral supplements are helpful but are difficult to take if you feel very sick. Eat the following foods to replenish vitamin and mineral levels:

✳ Wholemeal bread, chickpeas, seeds, hazelnuts and raisins, which are good sources of vitamin B^6.

✳ Milk, yogurt and white fish, which contain vitamin B^{12}.

✳ Green leafy vegetables, yeast extract, fortified breakfast cereals, nuts and pulses for folic acid.

✳ Broccoli, apricots and sardines to raise iron levels.

✳ Poultry, lean meat, sunflower seeds, wholemeal bread and wheatgerm to replenish zinc.

✳ Nuts, wholegrains, apricots and tofu for magnesium.

See pages 30–1 for further information

EASING NAUSEA

Try this gentle breathing exercise before each meal. Place one hand on your stomach and the other hand on your chest and focus on your stomach as you breathe deeply for five minutes.

KEY TIPS

Rest as much as possible

✳

Eat what your body tells you to and drink plenty of water

✳

Eat small, frequent meals

✳

Avoid fatty or spicy foods

✳

Keep a snack by your bed to eat before getting up in the morning

CAUTIONS

Drink plenty of fluids to avoid dehydration, signs of which include rapid pulse, furry tongue, bad-smelling breath and passing little urine. If you are experiencing persistent vomiting (*see pages 38–9*), consult your doctor.

COMPLEMENTARY TREATMENTS

Before using a complementary treatment, please read any **Cautions** and the relevant page references

ACUPUNCTURE

Needles are inserted into acupoints on your body, depending on the history and nature of your morning sickness. Between four and six weekly treatments may be needed.

✱ A practitioner may insert fine needles into the Pericardium 6 acupoint, located on your forearm, for between 15 and 20 minutes.

See pages 134–5 for further information

ACUPRESSURE

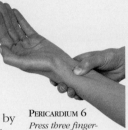

Based on the same Chinese principles as acupuncture – that sickness arises due to a blockage of *qi* – a practitioner balances *qi* by stimulating acupoints. Try these self-help measures:

PERICARDIUM 6
Press three finger-widths from the wrist, between both tendons.

✱ Stimulate the Pericardium 6 acupoint on your forearm to try to relieve nausea. Do this for ten minutes four times a day.

✱ Wear special acumagnets on the same acupoint day and night, since this can sometimes bring relief.

See page 136 for further information

REFLEXOLOGY

Nausea and sickness may respond to reflexology, especially in combination with other complementary treatments such as

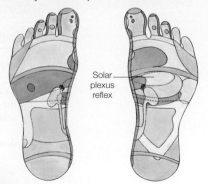

Solar plexus reflex

acupuncture, shiatsu or homeopathy. A reflexologist will gently massage the solar

plexus zone on the sole of the left foot that is linked to the relief of nausea.

See pages 140–1 for further information

YOGA & MEDITATION

Yoga and meditation can ease nausea by relaxing the diaphragm. To encourage relaxation, a yoga practitioner teaches a series of postures (*asanas*) that aim to integrate mind and body, so relieving tension.

✱ If any thoughts intrude during meditation, simply concentrate on the sensation of breathing.

See pages 142–3 for further information

WESTERN HERBALISM

Ginger is a key herb used in the treatment of morning sickness. It is rich in zinc, therefore helping to combat deficiency – a possible cause of nausea. It has been shown in clinical trials to reduce nausea and vomiting attacks.

✱ Eat ginger in any form, such as crystallized ginger or ginger biscuits, or, preferably, drink ginger tea. Infuse 5 g (1 tsp) grated ginger root in a cup of freshly boiled water for five minutes. Drink a cup two or three times a day or sip it frequently throughout the day.

✱ Other herbal teas can help, including chamomile, fennel, spearmint or peppermint. Drink a cup three times a day. Alternatively, any of these teas can be made into ice-cubes and sucked.

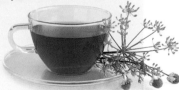

CHAMOMILE AND FENNEL
These gentle, soothing teas relieve sickness.

See pages 150–1 for further information

HOMEOPATHY

Try one of the following homeopathic self-help remedies, depending on your symptoms.

✱ For morning sickness with irritability, *Nux vomica 6c*.

✱ For inability to keep anything down but nausea not relieved by vomiting, *Ipecac. 6c*.

✱ For evening sickness and tearfulness, *Pulsatilla 6c*.

See pages 148–9 for dosage and further information

Hyperemesis

SEVERE VOMITING during pregnancy affects one in 100 women. Although not very common, it may well recur in subsequent pregnancies. Hyperemesis causes dehydration and upsets nutritional balance, and you may require hospitalization. Eating the right foods in the months prior to conception may help to prevent this condition.

SYMPTOMS

Inability to keep food down and severe, repeated vomiting

✳

Dehydration

✳

Side effect: depression and a feeling of isolation

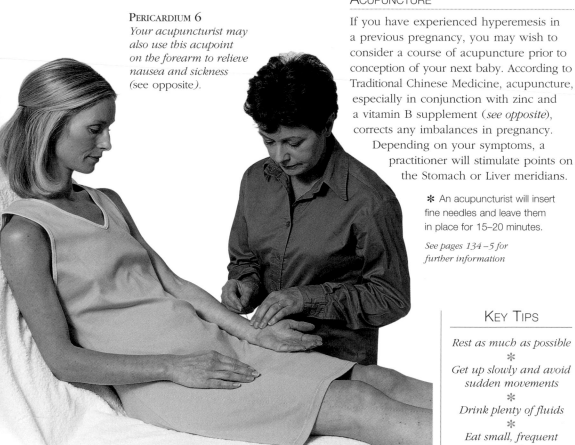

PERICARDIUM 6
Your acupuncturist may also use this acupoint on the forearm to relieve nausea and sickness (see opposite).

ACUPUNCTURE

If you have experienced hyperemesis in a previous pregnancy, you may wish to consider a course of acupuncture prior to conception of your next baby. According to Traditional Chinese Medicine, acupuncture, especially in conjunction with zinc and a vitamin B supplement (*see opposite*), corrects any imbalances in pregnancy. Depending on your symptoms, a practitioner will stimulate points on the Stomach or Liver meridians.

✳ An acupuncturist will insert fine needles and leave them in place for 15–20 minutes.

See pages 134–5 for further information

KEY TIPS

Rest as much as possible

✳

Get up slowly and avoid sudden movements

✳

Drink plenty of fluids

✳

Eat small, frequent snacks

✳

Avoid bad smells

✳

Have a bedtime snack to prevent blood sugar levels dropping at night

CAUTION

If you are experiencing persistent vomiting, watch for signs of dehydration (*see page 36*), continue to drink plenty of fluids and consult your doctor.

COMPLEMENTARY TREATMENTS

Before using a complementary treatment, please read any **Cautions** and the relevant page references

ACUPRESSURE

The Stomach and Liver meridians are often used in the treatment of nausea. In addition, the Pericardium 6 acupoint, located three finger-widths down the arm from the wrist crease, between the tendons, may be pressed for ten minutes four times a day to bring relief.

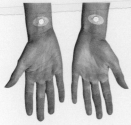

ACUMAGNETS
Sticky-backed acumagnets are easy to put in place.

✳ For the same effect, place acumagnets so that they put pressure on the Pericardium 6 acupoint.

✳ If you are very sick, use a TENS machine (*see page 109*). Place a pad on each Pericardium 6 acupoint for 45 minutes twice a day.

See page 136 for further information

CHIROPRACTIC

A chiropractor will manipulate your spine and joints in order to realign your body and improve digestive function. Studies have shown that this treatment can ease nausea.

See page 147 for further information

HYPNOTHERAPY

This treatment can help to alleviate stress and vomiting, but is only effective if you are receptive. Use a reputable practitioner who is recommended by the maternity services. A hypnotherapist may suggest self-help measures so that you can regulate the nausea at home.

See page 145 for further information

HOMEOPATHY

A homeopath will choose a remedy according to your symptoms. It might be:

✳ For sudden, spasmodic and severe vomiting, *Antim. tart. 6c*.

✳ For persistent vomiting that does not relieve the nausea, *Ipecac. 6c*.

See pages 148–9 for dosage and further information

AROMATHERAPY

You may find that burning essential oils such as lemon or bergamot in the room raises your spirits and relieves your nausea.

Caution: see page 153 for oils to avoid in pregnancy.

See pages 152–3 for further information

BERGAMOT
Fresh-smelling oil from the bergamot plant is uplifting.

FLOWER REMEDIES

Women with hyperemesis often feel anxious, tired and emotional. The following flower remedies may help to bring relief:

✳ Red chestnut if you are anxious about your baby.

✳ Crab apple for feelings of self-disgust.

✳ Chamomile for emotional upset.

See page 154 for further information

DIET & NUTRITION

The foetus can still obtain the nutrients it needs if you have hyperemesis, but try to eat the foods listed below. Bland carbohydrates, such as rice, baked potatoes, pasta and dry toast, however, may be the only foods you can tolerate. If you have had hyperemesis before, take a vitamin B^6 supplement before conceiving your next baby.

✳ Vitamin B^6 deficiency increases nausea. Eat bananas, chickpeas, wholemeal bread, brown rice and raisins.

✳ Pregnant women need extra zinc, and vegetarians often already lack zinc. Zinc-rich foods include ginger, poultry, lean meat, wholemeal bread and almonds.

✳ Magnesium is lost through vomiting, so eat plenty of nuts, wholegrains, wheatgerm and dried apricots.

✳ Potassium-rich foods, such as bananas, melons, raisins, figs and fruit juice, are essential after sickness.

See pages 30–1 for further information

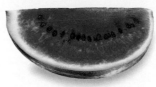

MELON
This fruit replenishes potassium, needed to redress fluid imbalance caused by vomiting.

Mouth Problems

HORMONAL CHANGES during pregnancy cause gums to thicken and soften, which may lead to tooth and gum problems. Gingivitis (inflamed gums) is common in the first half of pregnancy and can lead to bleeding gums and the loss of teeth. Cold sores on the lips are caused by the *herpes simplex* virus, and often appear if the immune system is weakened.

SYMPTOMS

Inflamed, sore and bleeding gums

✳

Blisters on the lips

✳

Unusual taste sensations

✳

Loose or aching teeth

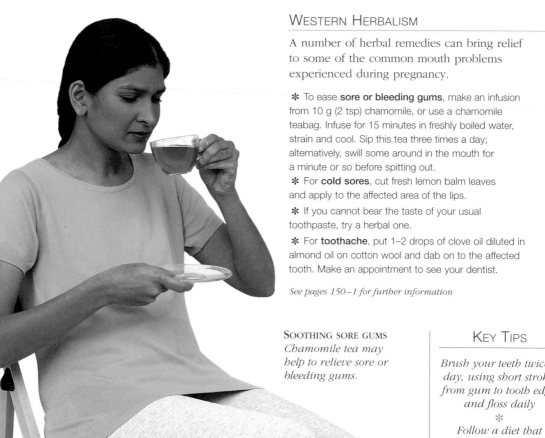

WESTERN HERBALISM

A number of herbal remedies can bring relief to some of the common mouth problems experienced during pregnancy.

✳ To ease **sore or bleeding gums**, make an infusion from 10 g (2 tsp) chamomile, or use a chamomile teabag. Infuse for 15 minutes in freshly boiled water, strain and cool. Sip this tea three times a day; alternatively, swill some around in the mouth for a minute or so before spitting out.

✳ For **cold sores**, cut fresh lemon balm leaves and apply to the affected area of the lips.

✳ If you cannot bear the taste of your usual toothpaste, try a herbal one.

✳ For **toothache**, put 1–2 drops of clove oil diluted in almond oil on cotton wool and dab on to the affected tooth. Make an appointment to see your dentist.

See pages 150–1 for further information

SOOTHING SORE GUMS
Chamomile tea may help to relieve sore or bleeding gums.

KEY TIPS

Brush your teeth twice a day, using short strokes from gum to tooth edge, and floss daily

✳

Follow a diet that is low in refined sugar and starch

✳

Have regular dental check-ups

✳

Use sunblock on the lips to help to prevent cold sores

CAUTION

Do not have mercury amalgam fillings replaced while you are pregnant in case mercury is released into your body.

COMPLEMENTARY TREATMENTS

Before using any complementary treatments, please read any **Cautions** and relevant page references

HOMEOPATHY

There are several homeopathic remedies that may be prescribed for ailments affecting the teeth, gums and lips. A homeopath can prescribe a constitutional remedy depending on your medical history and symptoms, or you can self-prescribe. Choose one of the following homeopathic remedies, depending to your specific symptoms:

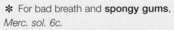

✳ For bad breath and **spongy gums**, *Merc. sol. 6c.*

✳ For red, inflamed, and **swollen gums** that bleed easily, *Kreosotum 6c.*

✳ For **bleeding gums**, *Phosphorus 6c.*

✳ For **cold sores**, *Natrum mur. 6c.*

PHOSPHORUS
Phosphorus is specifically prescribed for gums that bleed when touched.

See pages 148–9 for dosage and further information

DIET & NUTRITION

A varied diet that includes plenty of fresh fruit and vegetables – particularly green leafy vegetables – wholegrains, seeds and nuts, fish and lean meat will provide teeth and gums with all the nutrients that they need to stay healthy, and will boost the immune system so that it can fend off viruses. Be sure to chew food thoroughly, since the manipulation of food in the mouth helps to massage gums and increase blood flow through them. Your body's calcium requirement increases more than three-fold during pregnancy as the baby uses it to form teeth and bones. If your diet contains insufficient calcium, your baby's development may be affected and your own teeth and bones may also suffer as a result. It is also essential to eat foods that are good sources of magnesium, since this mineral

assists the absorption of calcium to create strong bones. Regular exercise also increases the absorption of calcium, as does vitamin D, which is produced under the skin by the action of ultraviolet radiation from the sun. Twenty minutes' exposure to the sun each day is probably all that you need. Make sure that you follow these dietary guidelines:

CITRUS FRUITS
A diet that is rich in fresh fruit will help to maintain healthy teeth and gums.

✳ Eat plenty of foods rich in vitamin C, which will maintain healthy gums and inhibit the development of **gingivitis**, **bleeding gums** and **cold sores**. Have five portions of fruit and vegetables daily; good choices are citrus fruit, blackcurrants, apples, apricots, cherries, Brussels sprouts, alfalfa, watercress and fresh parsley.

✳ Ensure that you receive sufficient calcium, which is essential for strong teeth, by eating parsley, watercress, nuts, sunflower seeds, eggs, low-fat milk, oily fish – for example, sardines and salmon – and chicken.

✳ Restrict intake of foods that inhibit calcium absorption. These include coffee, soft drinks, refined sugars, alcohol, protein (in excess) and salt.

✳ Eat foods that are rich in magnesium, which assists with calcium absorption. Good choices include dried apricots, wheatgerm, wholegrains, soya beans, cashew nuts, low-fat milk and yogurt.

✳ Include vitamin D-rich foods in your diet. Oily fish are by far the best source, but brown rice, eggs, milk, butter and margarine also contain vitamin D, which is needed to assist calcium absorption.

✳ Avoid eating large amounts of refined sugar and starch, since they can cause or exacerbate tooth decay while you have inflamed gums.

See pages 30–1 for further information

NUTS AND SEEDS
These are good sources of protein as well as of valuable nutrients such as magnesium.

Threatened Miscarriage

IT IS THOUGHT THAT ONE IN THREE PREGNANCIES miscarries; some women do not even realize they are pregnant. The causes of miscarriage include nutritional deficiencies, hormonal imbalance, infection, and auto-immune or chromosomal foetal disorders. Taking care prior to conception (*see pages 10–11*) is especially important if you have miscarried before.

ACUPUNCTURE

According to Traditional Chinese Medicine, the Kidneys are associated with reproduction. If there is weakness in the reproductive organs, an acupuncturist will aim to strengthen them by treating points on the Kidney meridian. The practitioner will take your case history, listen to your pulse and look at your tongue. Any sensations of heat or cold that you have are significant in cases of threatened miscarriage.

* The acupunture point that has traditionally been used in China in an attempt to prevent miscarriage is on the big toe (Sp 1). Moxa herb may be used to heat this point first.

SYMPTOMS

Backache

*

Abdominal cramping pains resembling period pains

*

Spots of blood or bleeding

KEY TIPS

Avoid alcohol

*

Avoid coffee, tea and cola drinks (caffeine has been linked to miscarriages)

*

Avoid hot baths

*

Do not smoke

*

Get plenty of rest, especially between 5 pm and 7 pm (see pages 132–3)

CAUTION

If you suspect that you might be about to miscarry, seek immediate medical attention. Therapies are only intended to complement, not replace, medical advice.

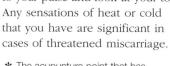
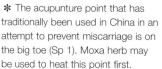

SPLEEN 1
A practitioner may heat the point on the big toe first – by lighting a small moxa cone with an akabani stick.

COMPLEMENTARY TREATMENTS

Before using a complementary treatment, please read any **Cautions** and the relevant page references

REST & RELAXATION

Depending on the severity of the risk, you may need to simply avoid strenuous activity (and not have sex); take a few hours of bed rest each day, lying on your side for some of the time to improve blood flow to the placenta; or lie down all day, getting up only to use the bathroom. Use meditation and deep breathing techniques to encourage profound relaxation.

VISUALIZATION

Concentrate on your baby in the uterus, sending positive thoughts to it. Also try to visualize the colour blue, regarded as the colour of healing. In Traditional Chinese Medicine, blue is related to the water element and to the Kidneys, which are believed to be responsible for reproduction. Try sitting quietly for 15 minutes, visualizing an area of blue around your lower back and abdomen.

See page 143 for further information

VISUALIZATION
The power of thought may help to promote healing and therefore prevent miscarriage.

HOMEOPATHY

Depending on your symptoms, a homeopath may prescribe one of the following remedies to prevent a threatened miscarriage:

✻ For a steady loss of bright red blood, cramping abdominal pain, weakness and nausea, *Ipecac. 30c.*

✻ For stitching pains that begin in the back and spread to the front, *Kali carb. 30c.*

✻ For intermittent loss of dark red blood which is more profuse each time it occurs, *Pulsatilla 30c.*

See pages 148–9 for dosage and further information

WESTERN HERBALISM

False unicorn root has traditionally been given to prevent miscarriage, but this must only be taken under careful supervision by a medical herbalist. Ginger can also taken to prevent miscarriage, either added to food or as a tea. To make ginger tea, grate 5 g (1 tsp) fresh ginger and infuse in a cup of freshly boiled water.

See pages 150–1 for further information

AROMATHERAPY

Burn either lavender or lemon essential oil in a vaporizer to promote relaxation and help to reduce the threat of miscarriage.

Caution: see page 153 for oils to avoid in pregnancy.

See pages 152–3 for further information

FLOWER REMEDIES

Flower remedies may help to reduce anxiety about threatened miscarriage.

✻ Mimulus combats anxiety.

✻ White chestnut alleviates worry.

✻ Sweet chestnut eases despair.

See page 154 for further information

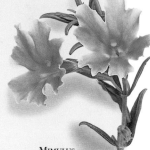

MIMULUS
The remedy made from this flower may dispel apprehension.

DIET & NUTRITION

Take multivitamins every day. Vitamin E may strengthen the placental link and reduce spotting, so take a supplement for two or three weeks or eat foods such as sweet potatoes and green leafy vegetables. Like vitamin E, selenium is an anti-oxidant and may help to prevent miscarriage. Take a supplement for three weeks or eat foods such as seafood or Brazil nuts.

✻ If you are bleeding, eat iron-rich foods, such as watercress and spinach, to prevent anaemia (see also pages 56–7).

See pages 30–1 for further information

GARLIC
Garlic is another source of the anti-oxidant selenium.

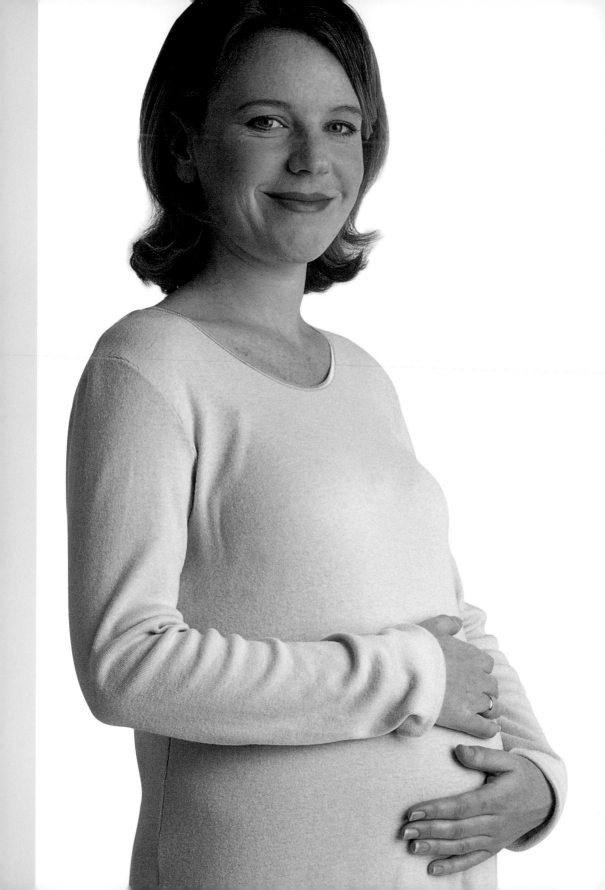

DURING THIS STAGE of your pregnancy you may well be "blooming", with shining hair and glowing skin. For many women this is the most enjoyable time: you should by now know the results of most antenatal tests and generally be feeling more confident and comfortable about your pregnancy. Sickness and exhaustion should

The second trimester

have lessened, while appetite and energy should have returned. There are some common problems and minor ailments that might affect you, however. This chapter offers practical advice to help you feel your best, both mentally and physically, and maintain a healthy diet and beneficial exercise programme.

Development of Mother & Baby

BY NOW YOU SHOULD BE LESS TIRED and your appetite should start to improve. You will notice the first signs of a "bump" as the uterus begins to grow rapidly. You will be more aware of the baby as an individual, which may encourage strong nurturing feelings.

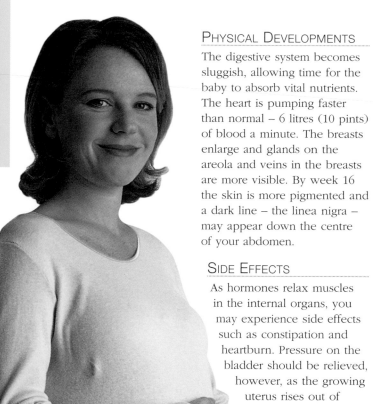

PHYSICAL DEVELOPMENTS

The digestive system becomes sluggish, allowing time for the baby to absorb vital nutrients. The heart is pumping faster than normal – 6 litres (10 pints) of blood a minute. The breasts enlarge and glands on the areola and veins in the breasts are more visible. By week 16 the skin is more pigmented and a dark line – the linea nigra – may appear down the centre of your abdomen.

SIDE EFFECTS

As hormones relax muscles in the internal organs, you may experience side effects such as constipation and heartburn. Pressure on the bladder should be relieved, however, as the growing uterus rises out of the pubic cavity. By week 18 your

LOOKING PREGNANT
You will have a noticeable "bump" and your waistline will have disappeared.

increased blood supply may cause nasal congestion and the occasional nosebleed. You may sweat more because of your increased metabolic rate. By week 17 you will be laying down fat: by week 24 you will be gaining 225–450 g (½–1 lb) a week in weight. This may increase further at week 27 as your baby puts on a growth spurt. The bump will be noticably bigger, and stretch marks may appear across your abdomen. The increased weight of the baby together with the softening affect of hormones on joints and ligaments will alter your sense of gravity.

AWARENESS OF BABY

By week 16 you may be aware of a "quickening" – the baby's first tangible movements. This feels like a slight fluttering or bubbling in your abdomen. By week 20, the baby's movements will be obvious. A couple of weeks later you will be able to detect cycles of activity and sleep. You may even be able to detect the baby's hiccups. By week 24, the baby may move when you start to speak.

THE BABY'S DEVELOPMENT

WEEK 13 The body is growing rapidly. The placenta now maintains the pregnancy, supplying nutrients and oxygen.

WEEK 14 The baby is aware of noise and light and responds to touch. Limbs are fully formed. Kidneys are beginning to function: the baby swallows amniotic fluid, rather than absorbing it through the skin, and excretes it. Few infections cross the placenta now.

WEEK 15 The body is growing faster than the head and movements are more vigorous. The bones still consist of soft cartilage but are beginning to ossify. Brain cells are increasing by 250,000 a minute.

WEEK 16 Facial features are looking more human. Fine hair (lanugo) is forming all over the body. Nerves are beginning to develop myelin sheaths, which will speed up neural connections.

WEEK 17 The baby measures about 18 cm (7 in) in length and weighs about 170 g (6 oz). The face can frown and squint; eyelashes and eyebrows are developing.

WEEK 18 The baby is practising breathing, taking amniotic fluid into the lungs and "breathing" it out again. It may have started to suck its thumb.

WEEK 19 Brain cells are continuing to multiply at an astonishing rate: between 50,000 and 100,000 a minute. The spinal cord is starting to thicken.

WEEK 20 The baby is roughly half as long as it will be at birth. Hair is growing on the head. Growth now slows, allowing body systems to mature.

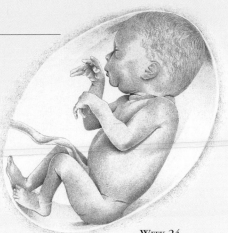

WEEK 24

WEEK 21 Taste buds have developed. The baby is starting to drink large amounts of amniotic fluid.

WEEK 22 Ears are fully formed. The baby may be able to learn and respond to sounds and voices. Music may stimulate brain-cell activity.

WEEK 23 Limbs are well developed and hands are able to grip. You will be able to identify different parts of the baby's body through the abdominal wall.

WEEK 24 Eyes can open. The baby can identify voices. Air sacs in the lungs are fully formed though, if born now, the baby would have severe breathing difficulties. All major organs are formed. Heart rate has dropped and is recordable. Skin is translucent and blood vessels clearly visible through it.

WEEK 25–26 Waking and sleeping periods established. The baby is covered in vernix, a white, greasy substance that nourishes, protects and waterproofs the skin.

WEEK 27 The baby is starting to put on weight as it begins another growth spurt. The amount of amniotic fluid increases.

SECOND TRIMESTER

Nutrition for Mother & Baby

By the second trimester, the nausea and extreme exhaustion of early pregnancy should be easing off. You will find that your energy levels increase and your appetite improves. Diet continues to be of great importance and certain nutrients are especially valuable at this stage of the baby's development.

FUELLING DEVELOPMENT

During the second trimester you will gain weight at the rate of about 450 g (1 lb) a week and your blood volume will increase. Progesterone will cause you to lay down fat to ensure there is enough "fuel" for milk production after the birth. The baby's development continues apace (*see page 47*). By the end of 14 weeks, its limbs are fully formed. By 21 weeks, the baby also will be laying down fat stores. Its nervous system is becoming more sophisticated and brain cells are multiplying at a staggering rate of at least 50,000 and 100,000 every minute. By the end of 24 weeks, the baby's other vital organs are maturing and the developing skeletal system is continuing to ossify.

KEY NUTRIENTS

Calcium is needed to form strong bones and teeth, to support muscle growth and to control nerve and muscle function in your baby. It is essential for you for blood clotting, and it may help to prevent raised blood pressure. Your need for calcium increases by a factor of at least three during pregnancy, although the ability of the body to absorb calcium becomes more efficient. Like calcium, phosphorus helps to form and maintain healthy bones and teeth. It is important for energy production and metabolism, and is needed for milk production. Magnesium is also essential for the baby's development, combining with calcium to build muscles, cells and nerves. It is needed for the functioning of the baby's liver and heart and for the metabolism of protein and carbohydrates.

KEY DAILY DIETARY CONSTITUENTS

7 servings of grains

6 servings of vegetables

4 servings of fruit, 2 of which are rich in vitamin C

3 servings of lean meat or pulses

3 servings of calcium-rich foods

3 servings of phosphorus-rich foods

3 servings of magnesium-rich foods

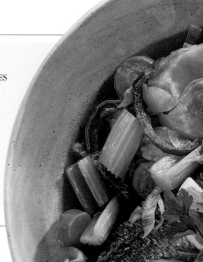

BAKED FISH WITH VEGETABLES *Fish such as grey mullet or bream, cooked with carrots, celery, peppers and garlic, supply protein and many nutrients.*

EXER...

1 KNEEL
*on you
knees.
the ba
your p
mirro*

2 PULL
MUSCL
*botto
the pe
breat
back
Hold
breat*

on your ab
side of the
deeply, the
your botto
pelvis upw
the abdom
the baby.
seconds, t
care not t

PREVENTA...

As part of
strengthen
exercise p
33) you c
that may

LEG CIRCLI
*Lift the foo
it outwar
large circ
the air. Re
with the o*

ESSENTIAL DIETARY NUTRIENTS

VITAMINS & MINERALS	FOR MOTHER	FOR BABY
VITAMIN A Half your intake of beta carotene may be converted into vitamin A.	*For maintaining immune system, healthy mucous membranes, bones, teeth, skin and hair.*	*For healthy neurons in the brain, cell membranes and vision.*
B VITAMINS Increased amounts are produced naturally in the body during pregnancy.	*B^6 and B^{12} to assist protein metabolism (extra protein is needed throughout pregnancy).*	*For development of nervous system, processing fatty acids and for energy.*
VITAMIN C This cannot be stored so regular intakes are necessary, but do not exceed 500 mg a day.	*For hormone production, boosting the immune system and iron absorption.*	*For collagen production, tissue growth, and healthy bones, teeth and skin.*
VITAMIN D The need for vitamin D increases throughout pregnancy, especially if not much time is spent outdoors.	*To store vitamin D to supply baby; for hormonal action and calcium and phosphate absorption.*	*For development of strong bones, especially foetal skull, and teeth.*
FOLATE The body stores very little folate so folic acid supplements will probably be needed.	*For hormonal action, protein metabolism, energy release, healthy nervous system.*	*For development of the nervous system, especially the spine.*
IRON The number of red blood cells in the body increases by 30 per cent during pregnancy.	*For haemoglobin production and prevention of anaemia.*	*For haemoglobin production.*
CALCIUM	*See* Key Nutrients, *opposite.*	*See* Key Nutrients, *opposite.*
PHOSPHORUS	*See* Key Nutrients, *opposite.*	*See* Key Nutrients, *opposite.*
MAGNESIUM	*See* Key Nutrients, *opposite.*	*See* Key Nutrients, *opposite.*

SUGGESTED MEAL PLAN

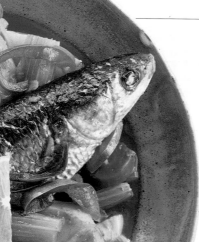

BREAKFAST
Cornflakes with sunflower seeds, banana and milk; wholemeal toast; orange juice

MIDMORNING SNACK
Walnuts and prunes

LUNCH
Wholemeal sandwich with salmon and avocado filling; kiwi fruit and a slice of melon

AFTERNOON SNACK
Houmous with carrot sticks

DINNER
Chicken stir-fry with beansprouts, ginger, baby corn, sesame seeds, mangetouts and brown rice

BEDTIME SNACK
Homemade popcorn

SECOND TRIMESTER

As far
is abo
muscl
mainta
group
physic

GENEF
You sh
aware
relating
pregna
It is es
warm
form o
down
(*see pa*

C

ST
Sto
ba
an
to
on
yo
su
do
fl

A
Be
w
do
be
fr
ed
th
th
w

THIRD TRIMESTER

Development of Mother & Baby

YOU MAY FEEL AS IF YOU HAVE BEEN PREGNANT for ever. At any time now you will start to produce colostrum and experience the first "practice" (Braxton Hicks) contractions, which are irregular and painless. Pelvic joints and ligaments are expanding ready for the birth.

KEY TIPS

See your midwife every two weeks from 29 weeks and every week from 36 weeks

✳

Rest as much as possible

✳

Monitor the baby's movements: if they seem to stop, consult your midwife

✳

Seek help for any urinary problems immediately

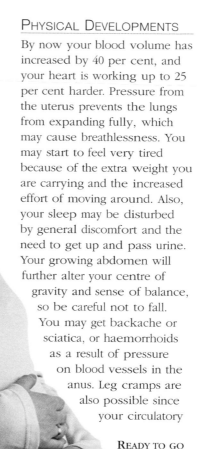

PHYSICAL DEVELOPMENTS

By now your blood volume has increased by 40 per cent, and your heart is working up to 25 per cent harder. Pressure from the uterus prevents the lungs from expanding fully, which may cause breathlessness. You may start to feel very tired because of the extra weight you are carrying and the increased effort of moving around. Also, your sleep may be disturbed by general discomfort and the need to get up and pass urine. Your growing abdomen will further alter your centre of gravity and sense of balance, so be careful not to fall. You may get backache or sciatica, or haemorrhoids as a result of pressure on blood vessels in the anus. Leg cramps are also possible since your circulatory system is working twice as hard as it usually does. By 32–33 weeks you will be gaining weight faster than at any other time in pregnancy. You will be feeling very heavy, having gained 8.5–11.25 kg (21–7 lb). Blood flow through the placenta has reached 450 litres (100 gal) a day. Overwork or lack of rest will impede this and affect the baby's growth.

READY FOR BIRTH

You should begin antenatal classes at about week 32. In 57 per cent of pregnancies the baby will turn after week 32 so that it is head-down; a further 25 per cent turn after week 36. At any time from then on the head will engage in the pelvis. Engagement is a preparation for labour but it does not mean that the birth is imminent. Some babies do not engage until after labour has begun. By week 37 weight gain will be slowing, although some women may suffer from water retention. By week 38 you will be feeling large and uncomfortable, and Braxton Hicks contractions may be strong and frequent.

READY TO GO
The abdomen changes shape once the baby is in a head-down position and ready to be born.

THE BABY'S DEVELOPMENT

WEEK 28 Eyes are open sometimes and developing the ability to focus. If born now the baby would, with special care, have a good chance of survival. A boy's testes now descend into the groin.

WEEK 29 The baby is about 34 cm (13½ in) in length and covered with vernix. The lungs have developed most of their alveoli and are producing surfactant, a wetting agent, to assist breathing.

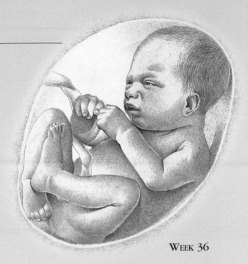

WEEK 36

WEEK 30 During several weeks of moving around, the baby has increased muscle tone and developed the ability to orientate itself in space. Very occasionally it will turn so that it is in a head-down position.

WEEK 31 The skin is becoming pink rather than red as a result of the white fat deposits that have been laid down beneath it. These will provide energy and regulate temperature after the baby is born.

WEEK 32 The vernix is very thick and there may be quite a lot of hair on the head. Fingernails are fully grown but toenails are not. The face is smooth by now with few wrinkles.

WEEK 33 The baby is almost completely formed and in the proportions you would expect to see at birth. It is gaining weight. The body systems are still maturing.

WEEK 34 The brain and nervous system are fully developed. The immune system is still immature and the baby continues to receive its mother's antibodies. It is about 37 cm (15 in) in length.

WEEK 35 The baby's movements may start to slow down now as there is less room to manoeuvre.

WEEK 36 Seventy per cent of the oxygen and nutrients coming through the placenta are used by the brain. If the baby were born now, it would be mature enough to survive without too many problems. More fat is accumulating under the skin. Meconium, a dark green, thick substance made up of dead cells and secretions from the bowel and liver, is being produced in the intestines.

WEEK 37 The baby will be practising breathing, sucking and swallowing. Its level of consciousness and degree of co-ordination will by this stage be well established.

WEEK 38 The baby is ready to be born. (Its development has taken 38 weeks from the moment of conception. Forty weeks of pregnancy is calculated from the first day of your last menstrual period.) The baby is plump and only just fits inside the uterus. It has to curl up tightly. The head will now descend into the lower part of the uterus and press through the softened, partially opened cervix, ready for the birth.

THIRD TRIMESTER

Nutrition for Mother & Baby

THERE ARE, AS IN THE FIRST TWO TRIMESTERS, windows of nutritional opportunity during the last three months of pregnancy. This period includes the time when you should be preparing your body for giving birth (*see also pages 98–9*), but also providing sustenance for crucial brain growth in your baby prior to the birth.

(*see also pages 98–9*)

KEY TIPS

Make sure that the fats in your diet are mainly polyunsaturated

✳

Include plenty of foods rich in iron and vitamin C in your diet

✳

Eat plenty of "brain foods"

FUELLING DEVELOPMENT

Your blood volume is still increasing, so you need plenty of iron-rich foods as well as vitamin C for good absorption of the iron. You are gaining weight faster than at any other time in the pregnancy, laying down fat ready for producing milk. It is important to eat the right kind of fat – that is, polyunsaturated – to obtain essential fatty acids.

CRUCIAL BRAIN FOOD

The baby's brain is growing faster than ever. The number of brain cells is increasing at a rate of at least 100,000 a minute. Seventy per cent of the calories your baby receives are used for brain growth. When the baby is born, its brain weighs about 350 g (12 oz). Sixty per cent of it is made up of fat, and 20 per cent of that is composed of long-chain polyunsaturated fatty acids (LCPs). These "essential" fatty acids are required for the rapid transmission of signals between nerve cells. There are two kinds of essential fatty acids, both essential for good brain function: linoleic acid (omega–6) and linolenic acid (omega–3). The best food sources of omega–6 are seeds and their oils. The best sources of omega–3 are linseed, pumpkin seeds and oily fish. One of the active forms of omega–3 is DHA (docosahexaenoic acid), which is a component of brain-cell membranes and ensures good neural connections. There is evidence that DHA may help to prevent pregnancy-induced hypertension (raised blood pressure), and that it reduces the risk of premature birth, increases a baby's birth weight, improves its IQ and visual and cognitive brain function and also protects against heart disease.

KEY DAILY DIETARY CONSTITUENTS

7 servings of grains
6 servings of vegetables
4 servings of fruit, 2 of which are rich in vitamin C
3 servings of lean meat, fish or pulses
2 servings of calcium-rich food
1 serving of magnesium-rich food

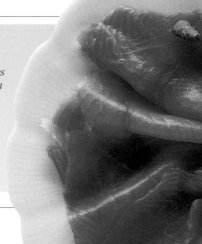

SMOKED SALMON SALAD
The fish provides valuable protein ready for labour and breastfeeding; the salad is light yet nutritious.

ESSENTIAL DIETARY NUTRIENTS

NUTRIENTS	FOR MOTHER	FOR BABY
VITAMIN A This is a powerful anti-oxidant.	*For production of hormones for lactation and good immunity.*	*For maintaining healthy mucous membranes.*
B VITAMINS Vitamins B2 is needed in increased amounts as well as those listed (*see For Mother, right*).	*B^1 for energy production; B^6 for protein metabolism; folate to make DNA and (with B^{12}) to make red blood cells.*	*B^1 for energy production.*
VITAMIN E This is a powerful anti-oxidant.	*Speeds up wound healing; increases skin suppleness; may strengthen uterine muscles.*	*For development of the nervous system and heart.*
OTHER VITAMINS K is made naturally in the gut, but not in a baby's, so it may be given orally at birth.	*C for iron absorption, hormone production, and resistance to infection; K for blood clotting.*	*K for blood clotting.*
CALCIUM Foetus takes up calcium at a rate of about 350 mg a day.	*For prevention of pre-eclampsia and raised blood pressure; (with vitamin D) to ease labour pains.*	*For development of bones and teeth.*
ZINC Boys take five times as much zinc as girls: deficiency is linked to undescended testes.	*For hormonal balance; may help to prevent stretch marks.*	*For development and growth of reproductive system.*
OTHER MINERALS Iron intake must be kept high because it takes six weeks to build up supplies.	*Iron for manufacture of red blood cells (vitamins C, B^6, B^{12} and folate improve absorption).*	*Selenium for brain development; phosphorus for bone development.*

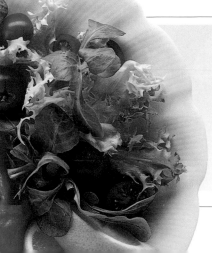

SUGGESTED MEAL PLAN

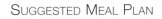

BREAKFAST
Branflakes and raisins with milk; sardines and grilled tomatoes on wholemeal toast; grapefruit juice

MIDMORNING SNACK
Fruit milkshake

LUNCH
Broccoli and sunflower seed soup; wholemeal turkey and watercress sandwich; peach

AFTERNOON SNACK
Watermelon juice; ten cashew nuts and a banana

DINNER
Carrot juice; wholewheat pasta with meat/lentil bolognese and grated cheese; rocket and walnut salad

BEDTIME SNACK
Rest of broccoli soup with wholemeal bread and butter

THIRD TRIMESTER

Sleeplessness

SLEEPING DIFFICULTIES are common during pregnancy and lead to fatigue during the day. In early pregnancy, low blood sugar levels as a result of hunger or nausea may cause insomnia. As pregnancy progresses, many women are unable to relax fully in bed due to general discomfort, heartburn, leg cramps or worry about the baby.

SYMPTOMS

Difficulty in falling asleep

*

Restless, unrefreshing sleep with periods of wakefulness

*

Fatigue and irritability during the day

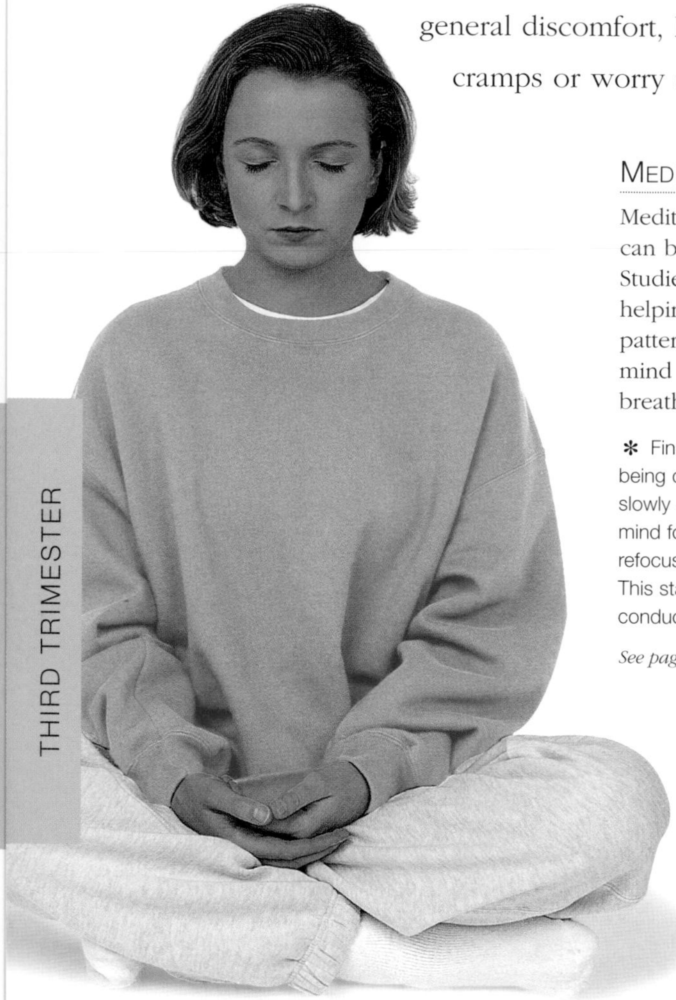

MEDITATION

Meditation, particularly Transcendental Meditation, can be used to induce a state of deep relaxation. Studies show that meditation focuses the mind, helping to lower blood pressure, improve brainwave patterns and so encourage sleep. Try to clear your mind of all other matters and focus only on your breathing. Use the following technique:

* Find a quiet place where you can meditate without being disturbed. Make yourself comfortable and breathe slowly and regularly for 30 minutes. Try to keep your mind focused on your breathing patterns, and gently refocus your attention if your mind starts to wander. This state of "passive awareness" will make you more conducive to sleep.

See page 143 for further information

POSE FOR THOUGHT
Meditation allows you to concentrate your thoughts in order to calm the mind, relieve tension and induce sleep.

KEY TIPS

Relax before bed and avoid mental stimulation

*

Try to take regular exercise each day

*

Avoid drinks containing caffeine in the evening

*

Eat a substantial lunch and a light supper

*

Eat calcium and magnesium-rich foods, thought to calm nerves

THIRD TRIMESTER

CAUTION

If sleeplessness persists for longer than two weeks, consult your midwife or doctor because persistent sleep deprivation alters mood.

COMPLEMENTARY TREATMENTS

Before using a complementary treatment, please read any **Cautions** and the relevant page references

ACUPUNCTURE

A practitioner will require details of your sleep patterns. If you cannot sleep between 11 pm and 1 am for example, the peak time for the Gall Bladder meridian, acupuncture points along this meridian will be stimulated to correct any imbalance. Dream-disturbed sleep will also be of interest to a practitioner, since this may indicate a disturbed spirit, or *shen*. Research shows that acupuncture helps to increase production of the neurotransmitter serotonin, which is sometimes deficient in people who have sleeping problems.

See pages 134–5 for further information

SHIATSU

Insomnia is regarded as a disturbance of *shen* (*see above*), and is associated with the Heart meridian. Stimulating the Heart 7 acupoint, located on the inside of the wrists, can help to combat sleeplessness. Apply pressure to the point for 10–15 seconds before you go to bed.

INSOMNIA ACUPOINT
To locate Heart 7, run your finger down from the tip of your little finger to the wrist crease.

See page 138 for further information

WESTERN HERBALISM

There are many herbal teas available that help to relax the nervous system. They include chamomile and lemon balm. Steep a teabag in a cup of freshly boiled water for 10 minutes and drink before bed.

See pages 150–1 for further information

HOME-MADE TEA BAG
To make a tea bag, put 5–10 g (1–2 tsp) dried herbs in a muslin square and secure with string.

AROMATHERAPY

Lavender essential oil, added to a bath or to a carrier oil for massage, can help you to relax. Ask your partner to massage your neck and shoulders gently before you go to bed.

❋ Burn lemon or mandarin oil in a vaporizer; in Traditional Chinese Medicine, mandarin is used to calm the spirit.

Caution: see page 153 for oils to avoid in pregnancy.

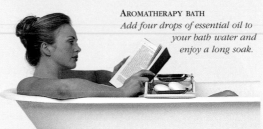

AROMATHERAPY BATH
Add four drops of essential oil to your bath water and enjoy a long soak.

See pages 152–3 for further information

FLOWER REMEDIES

If sleeplessness is due to anxiety, flower remedies may help. Take two drops twice a day in a cup of water, and again before bed. Choice of remedy will depend on symptoms.

❋ Rock rose for any terrifying thoughts.

❋ White chestnut for niggling worries.

❋ Red chestnut to free the mind of negative, fearful thoughts and worries about your baby.

See page 154 for further information

DIET & NUTRITION

Vitamin B deficiency may cause insomnia. If blood sugar levels fall during the night, you may wake because of hunger or nausea.

❋ Calcium-rich foods help to induce sleep by calming the nerves. Eat foods such as almonds, yogurt or sesame seeds as evening snacks.

❋ Foods rich in vitamin B6, such as pulses, green leafy vegetables, nuts, wholegrains and meat have a tranquilizing effect.

See pages 72–3 for further information

THIRD TRIMESTER

Respiratory Problems

FROM EARLY PREGNANCY, the lungs and diaphragm become compressed in order to accommodate the expanding uterus. Breathing becomes shallower, and any respiratory weakness, such as a tendency to hayfever, may worsen. You may also find yourself more prone to respiratory infections, which can be exacerbated by a poor diet that is full of additives.

SYMPTOMS

Streaming eyes, running or blocked nose

✳

Sore throat, hoarseness, loss of voice, cough

✳

Breathing difficulties, fever, pain

INHALATING VAPOURS
Essential oils, inhaled in steam, can ease respiratory problems. A towel over the head helps to trap the steam.

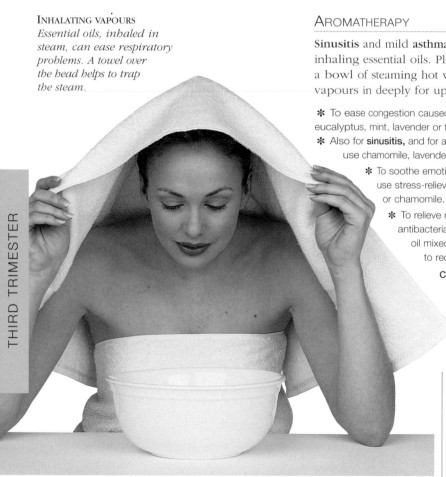

AROMATHERAPY

Sinusitis and mild **asthma** may be relieved by inhaling essential oils. Place four drops of oil in a bowl of steaming hot water, then breathe the vapours in deeply for up to 15 minutes.

✳ To ease congestion caused by **sinusitis**, use eucalyptus, mint, lavender or tea tree essential oils.
✳ Also for **sinusitis,** and for allergy-induced **asthma,** use chamomile, lavender or sandalwood.
✳ To soothe emotionally-induced **asthma**, use stress-relieving neroli, lavender, rose, or chamomile.
✳ To relieve respiratory infections, use antibacterial oils such as tea tree. This oil mixed with chamomile will help to reduce inflammation.

Cautions: only use pure oils; inhalation of some oils may exacerbate asthma; see page 153 for essential oils to avoid in pregnancy.

See pages 152–3 for further information

KEY TIPS

Eat plenty of oily fish, nuts and seeds

✳

Eat a variety of fresh fruit and vegetables daily

✳

Cut down on animal fats and dairy products

✳

Avoid foods laden with additives, preservatives or artificial colourants

CAUTIONS

Consult your doctor before taking natural remedies for asthma. Do not stop taking prescribed medication. For bronchitis, see your doctor immediately.

COMPLEMENTARY TREATMENTS

Before using a complementary treatment, please read any **Cautions** and the relevant page references

ACUPUNCTURE

In Traditional Chinese Medicine, **hayfever** is regarded as an invasion of "heat" and "wind", and can be treated at acupoints on the back. Treating points on the Lung and Kidney meridians may help those with **asthma**.

See pages 134–5 for further information

YOGA

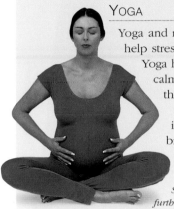

Yoga and meditation can help stress-related **asthma**. Yoga has an overall calming effect, while the controlled stretching postures it uses can improve breathing control and help to expand the lungs.

See page 142 for further information

DEEP BREATHING
Sitting comfortably and concentrating on deep breathing induces calm and improves technique.

ALEXANDER TECHNIQUE

The improved posture taught by an Alexander teacher may reduce the shoulder hunching that is common to many people with **asthma**.

See page 147 for further information

HOMEOPATHY

A number of self-help remedies can be used to treat **hayfever**, depending on the precise nature of your symptoms:

✽ For burning eyes, frequent sneezing, runny nose, puffy eyelids and exhaustion, *Arsen. alb. 6c.*

✽ For burning nasal **catarrh**, sneezing and eye inflammation, *Allium cepa 6c.*

✽ For itchy ears, stuffy nose, inflamed eyes and watery catarrh, *Euphrasia 6c.*

✽ For chronic **rhinitis**, *Nux vomica. 6c.*

See pages 148–9 for dosage and further information

WESTERN HERBALISM

A number of herbs help to relieve respiratory problems. Steep 5–10 g (1–2 tsp) dried herb in 250 ml (9 fl oz) freshly boiled water for about 10 minutes, then drink. Take three times a day. Some herbs can be used in cooking.

✽ To ease **asthma**, try ginger, German chamomile, elderflower, nettle or thyme. Capsules of evening primrose oil may help some types of asthma, particularly if it is allergy-related.

✽ To soothe **bronchitis**, use thyme or ginger. Garlic and onions, eaten raw if possible, have good antibacterial properties.

✽ To clear **catarrhal** congestion, sip elderflower tea or 1 tbsp (15 ml) cider vinegar in hot water. Alternatively, make an infusion of thyme.

✽ To ease mild **hayfever**, drink tea made from chamomile, lavender, nettle, or take dandelion root tincture.

See pages 150–1 for further information

DIET & NUTRITION

Oily fish are rich in omega-3 fatty acids, which may alleviate inflammation and allergic reactions. Vitamin E and selenium are good anti-inflammatories, and are found in cold-pressed oils, green leafy vegetables, nuts and sunflower seeds. Vitamin C (found in foods such as broccoli, tomatoes, peppers and citrus fruit) is an antihistamine. Follow these other dietary guidelines:

✽ To prevent respiratory ailments from being exacerbated by dairy products, limit your intake but supplement your diet with calcium-rich alternatives such as sesame seeds, broccoli, tofu, sardines or watercress.

✽ To ease **asthma**, eliminate foods that you are allergic to while maintaining a balanced diet. In general, lower your fat intake and increase your fish and fruit consumption.

✽ To relieve severe **hayfever**, take vitamin C and pantothenic acid supplements.

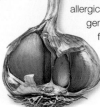

See pages 72–3 for further information

Countdown to Labour

IN THE LAST FEW WEEKS before your baby is born it will help you mentally to know that you are taking positive steps towards the event. It is not easy to think beyond labour, especially if this is your first baby and you are, understandably, feeling apprehensive.

Rest as much as possible

✳

Eat what your body tells you to and drink plenty of fresh water

THE LAST FEW WEEKS OF PREGNANCY

WEEK 34

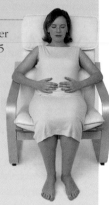

✳ You will have started antenatal classes.
✳ Make sure you have an adequate night's sleep and two hours' rest in the afternoon.
✳ Exercise three times a week to suit you (*see pages 18–19 and 74–5*).
✳ Visualize your baby and communicate positive thoughts (*see right and page 143*).
✳ Eat iron-rich foods (*see pages 13*).
✳ Daily massage of the perineum before the birth may help to prevent tears. Soak in a bath to soften the area. Place natural plant oil on your thumb or index finger and place in the vagina at least 5 cm (2 in), pressing towards the rectum. Gently stretch the area in a U-shaped motion until you feel a tingling sensation. Release and massage. Repeat for five to ten minutes.
✳ Start taking raspberry leaf, either as tea or tablets, to help to tone the uterus.

WEEK 35

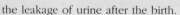

✳ Go over the Shiatsu points for labour with your partner.
✳ Do some pelvic floor exercises (*see page 75*) every day. Toning the muscles of the pelvic floor will help them to stretch and recoil more easily during and after the birth, and will also help to prevent the leakage of urine after the birth.
✳ Exercise gently for a little while every day. Swimming, walking and yoga are good at this stage.
✳ Practise gentle stretching that will help to prepare your pelvis for labour, such as tailor sitting (*see left and page 74*).

WEEK 36

✳ You may start to feel fed up with being pregnant, especially if you are tired, uncomfortable and sleeping badly. Have a relaxing aromatherapy massage.
✳ Mugwort flower remedy may encourage the baby to engage (*see page 154*).
✳ Try olive flower remedy if you are exhausted, hornbeam if you are doubting your ability to cope or mimulus if you are beginning to feel afraid.
✳ For an uplifting effect, use frankincense or lemon oil in a vaporizer (*see pages 152–3*).

Week 37

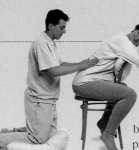

✻ Labour could happen at any time, and you may be feeling anxious. Keep practising your relaxation techniques.

✻ Rest is more important than ever. Put your feet up for a couple of hours during the day and make sure that you go to bed early.

✻ Practise massage techniques with a partner.

✻ Take vitamin C and zinc, both necessary for hormone production prior to delivery.

Week 38

✻ Start to eat a diet that is rich in carbohydrates (*see pages 98–9*).

✻ In the ten days before your due date, take the homeopathic remedy *Caulophylum 30c* each night before you go to bed for a week and *Caulophylum 200c* for the last three days. This will help to relieve the pain of contractions. It is best to consult a homeopath (*see pages 148–9*).

✻ Increase your intake of raspberry leaf tea to four cups a day.

✻ Eat plenty of magnesium- and calcium-rich foods to fortify the muscles ready for contractions during labour.

Week 39

✻ Co-enzyme Q10 improves the ability of muscles cells to use oxygen and metabolize energy (*see page 99*). Take as a supplement or eat rich food sources.

✻ Eat plenty of foods rich in vitamin K, which is vital for blood clotting (*see page 98*) for you and the baby.

✻ Start taking the homeopathic remedy *Arnica 6c* to help to prevent bruising after the birth (*see pages 148–9*).

Week 40

✻ Delivery should be any day now. Start to use acupressure (*see page 136*) and/or a TENS machine (*see page 109*) daily on acupoints LI 4 on the hand (to relieve anxiety and abdominal discomfort) and Sp 6 on the lower leg (to reduce haemorrhaging and strengthen the uterus) ready for labour.

✻ Drink fennel tea to increase milk flow ready for breastfeeding.

✻ Continue to practise positions for labour.

✻ Rest when you can and use the time to practise relaxation techniques (*see below*).

RELAXATION
Prop yourself up and support your knees with pillows when you lie on your back. Do not lie flat on your back at this stage of pregnancy, as this might restrict oxygen supply to the baby.

Nutrition during Labour

YOU SHOULD PREPARE YOURSELF FOR LABOUR as if you were in training for a marathon – at least in terms of energy requirements. Building up energy ready for labour will help to prevent tiredness, dehydration, weakness and demoralization, all of which increase the likelihood of medical intervention in the birth.

KEY NUTRIENTS

During the last few weeks of pregnancy you should build on the preceding months of healthy eating so that you are prepared for the rigours of labour. Vitamin K is needed in particular to control blood clotting, prevent haemorrhaging and help to heal the placental site. It is derived naturally from bacteria in the mother's gut and supplemented from rich food sources such as broccoli, beans, spinach, avocado, watercress, lettuce, cabbage and cauliflower. A baby's gut is sterile, however, so an infant depends on its mother for vitamin K, before birth via the placenta and after

through breast milk. (Babies may be given vitamin K orally at birth.) Zinc is another very important mineral in the run-up to labour. It is needed to encourage hormone production and healing after the birth.

PRODUCING ENERGY

Simple carbohydrates, which are basic sugars, are quickly absorbed from the digestive system into the bloodstream. Excess glucose in the blood is stored as glycogen in the liver and muscles. When cells need energy, they use the glucose in the blood. If the blood sugar level is low, energy is obtained from glycogen – the longterm

energy reserve. To maintain energy levels, you need to keep your blood sugar level constant by eating complex carbohydrates, which break down gradually and release their sugar content slowly. To ensure that glycogen reserves are filled to capacity, stock up on complex carbohydrates during the two weeks before the birth. This means eating lots of vegetables, wholegrains and pulses. In addition to complex carbohydrates, certain enzymes are needed for energy production. These in turn are dependant on vitamins and minerals. If these are deficient, you will not maximize your

ESSENTIAL DIETARY NUTRIENTS

| B vitamins, including folate |
| Vitamin C |
| Iron |
| Calcium |
| Magnesium |
| Zinc |
| Chromium |

VEGETABLE SOUP
You may not feel like a full meal as you approach labour, but a "big soup" – with a variety of vegetables, beans and ham in this case – is very nutritious.

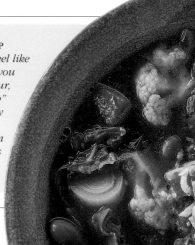

energy potential. To convert glucose into energy, you need:
- B vitamins (B[1], B[2], B[3], B[4], B[6], B[12]). Sources: meat, poultry, milk, eggs, vegetables, watercress, pulses, nuts, wholegrains. B vitamins include folate. Sources: broccoli, spinach, wheatgerm, seeds, nuts.
- Vitamin C. Sources: citrus fruit, blackcurrants, peppers, broccoli, tomatoes.
- Iron. Sources: pumpkin seeds, prunes, nuts, parsley, apricots.
- Choline, an organic substance needed for the transmission of signals between muscles and nerves during energy production. Sources: eggs, fish, soya beans, wholegrains, nuts, pulses.
- Calcium and magnesium, for maximizing the efficiency of contractions during labour. Sources: cheese, milk, parsley, seeds, beans, nuts, raisins.
- Chromium, for maintaining balanced blood sugar levels. Sources: potatoes, wholemeal bread, peppers, eggs, chicken.
- Co-enzyme Q10, for energy metabolism and the efficient use of oxygen by muscle cells. Sources: meat, fish, eggs, soya beans, spinach, broccoli, alfalfa.

FUEL DURING LABOUR

Until recently it was common practice not to eat or drink during labour in case medical intervention requiring the use of anaesthetic was necessary. Anaesthetic carries with it the risk of Mendelson's syndrome, whereby food may be regurgitated and acidic gastric juices inhaled, causing the potentially fatal respiratory distress syndrome. Feeling hungry and thirsty during labour, however, can also have detrimental effects. A lack of energy can slow down the progress of labour, reducing the efficiency of uterine contractions and making medical intervention more likely. If carbohydrates are not available and blood glucose and glycogen supplies are depleted, ketones begin to be produced as the body metabolizes fat stores. Ketones are organic substances that make blood more acidic and less able to transport oxygen efficiently. If you do not drink plenty of fluids during labour then you may become dehydrated, which will also

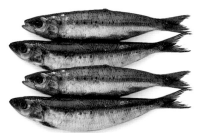

SARDINES
These fish are a good source of protein, calcium and other valuable nutrients.

adversely affect your energy levels. At worst, you may need an intravenous drip, which will greatly restrict your movements during labour. Ideally, you need an energy drink that is specifically designed for the extraordinary demands made upon your body during the often long hours of labour (isotonic sports drinks are not recommended). A combination of maltodextrin and fructose will ensure a sustained energy release, with glucose instantly available and a supply of micronutrients to help your body to metabolize energy efficiently. There are some specially formulated drinks available for this purpose.

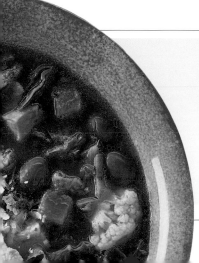

FOODS TO FUEL LABOUR

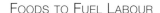

SMALL MEALS & SNACKS
- Small jacket potato
- Sandwiches
- Sardines on toast
- Cold pasta salad
- Rice salad
- Tabbouleh
- Bowl of cereal
- Dried fruit such as apricots
- Banana
- Apple and orange segments

- Grapes
- Celery sticks
- Cheese and biscuits
- Carrot sticks
- Bread sticks
- Crackers
- Cereal bars
- Nuts and raisins

Preparing the Mind

YOUR FRAME OF MIND can greatly enhance the progress of your labour and help to alleviate pain. The more relaxed you are the better. Mental preparation, for which you need adequate time, also helps you to adjust quicker to life after the birth. This is especially important if you are expecting your first baby.

PREPARATION TIME

Given the choice, most women would probably opt for time off after their baby is born rather than in the run-up to the birth. Working until just before the birth, however, means that you might go into labour mentally unprepared and physically exhausted, and it might take far longer to adjust and recover after the birth. Although pregnancy technically lasts for 40 weeks, labour may begin any time after 37 weeks, and giving up work at 32–34 weeks is highly recommended.

VOICING CONCERNS

If this is your first baby, or if you have had a difficult time with a previous birth, you may view labour with a great deal of apprehension. You may have specific fears about tearing, coping with pain or a general fear of the unknown or of something being wrong with the baby. It is important to admit to these fears and try to deal with them in advance, so that during labour you only have to think about what is actually happening to you.

BUILDING CONFIDENCE

Fear can slow your labour right down. Remember that a woman's body is designed for childbirth. The pelvis is the right shape to allow a baby to pass through, and the ligaments are built to stretch. So start your labour from a position of confidence and positive thoughts. Think of your birth plan as an action plan! Assemble your complementary therapies

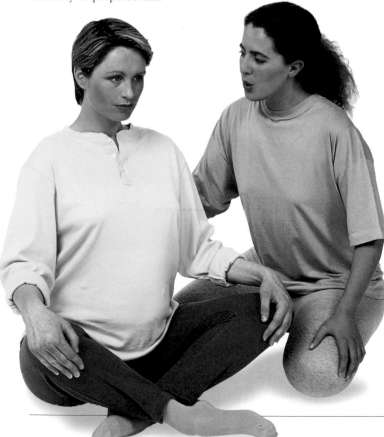

ANTENATAL CLASSES
These give you and your birth partner the opportunity to practise working as a team.

and plan with your partner which should be used when. Mark up acupressure points, practise using a TENS machine (*see page 109*) and make sure you are comfortable in the positions that you would like to adopt during labour and birth. Take note of the patterns of behaviour that you may develop during labour so that neither of you will be alarmed if they happen. Do not persuade a male partner to be with you during labour against his will. Support is obviously of great value but not if your partner is reluctant and feels pressurized. This will lead to feelings of inadequacy and possible tension between you later. Consider asking a close female friend instead, or anyone who you feel you can trust to give you the support you need.

MEDITATION & VISUALIZATION

Try to find a little time every day to sit quietly alone and clear your mind. Make yourself comfortable, close your eyes and focus on your breathing. Inhale and exhale slowly and naturally: just observe how you breathe rather than trying to change it. This is a wonderfully simple way to harmonize body, mind and spirit. After a few minutes, continue breathing naturally but consider the exhalation to be the start of the breathing cycle, rather than the inhalation. Imagine the kind of labour that you would like to have. Visualize positions you will adopt, the way in which you will cope with contractions, whether you would like a therapist with you, the way the

cervix will open, the way your baby will descend down the birth canal. Above all, imagine it to be a positive experience.

THE HEART-UTERUS CONNECTION

The Chinese believe that, when a woman becomes pregnant, a direct channel of communication opens up between her heart and that of the baby. It is important that any concerns, fears and vulnerabilities that the mother has are dealt with. The strength of her heart and spirit helps to establish a strong bond with the baby. The acupoint that is used to strengthen this link is Heart 7, which is located on the inside of the wrist crease and has physical, mental and emotional significance. The Heart blood is regarded as the house of your spirit and the seat of all emotions. If your blood is low (that is, you are anaemic), you may become low in spirits, depressed and tearful. The Chinese also believe that *qi*, or life energy, which flows throughout the body, can be improved by focusing the mind, inducing a state of deep relaxation and encouraging positive thought.

THE VALUE OF YOGA

Yoga uses postures and breathing techniques to improve physical health and mental well-being (*see page 142*). It is important to strengthen the Heart *chakra* prior to labour, so that you are emotionally strong and you feel able to

cope with anything, rather than being nervous and vulnerable. There are techniques, drawing on these similar traditional beliefs, that can be used to prepare you mentally in the run-up to labour.

• Sit cross-legged on the floor. Rub your hands vigorously against your thighs to create heat in the palms. Place the right palm over the lower abdomen, covered by the left hand. Imagine that the baby is

ALTERNATE NOSTRIL BREATHING
This deep-breathing technique can be used to induce a state of calm (see also page 66).

lying beneath your hands. Slide your right hand out and place it, palm down, on the sacrum (at the back of the pelvis), with the left hand still in place.

• Alternatively, slide the back of both wrists up and down the kidney area of the lower back to help to prepare for delivery of the baby.

Natural Pain Relief

MANY WOMEN PREFER NOT TO USE DRUGS to deal with the pain of labour. If you are expecting your first baby, you may not know how much pain you can tolerate. Knowledge of various methods of pain relief will give you confidence and help you to develop a positive attitude to pain as a means of getting the baby born.

KEY TIPS

Familiarize yourself with all the options for pain relief

✳

Give yourself time to prepare mentally

✳

Understand the physical effects of fear and anxiety

EFFECTS OF FEAR

It is important to appreciate the effects of fear on your labour. If you are frightened and in pain, the body releases the hormone adrenaline, producing the "fight or flight" response. Your circulatory, respiratory, genito-urinary, gastrointestinal and skeletal systems are all affected, resulting in increased blood sugar levels and heart rate, raised blood pressure and slower digestion. You will become agitated, the pain will increase and the progress of labour will be slowed. You should aim to feel as comfortable and secure as possible, happy in your environment and with the people who are supporting you.

THE BODY'S RESPONSE

The release of oxytocin shapes your contractions during labour. The hormone is produced as a result of pressure from the baby's head on the cervix: the greater the pressure, the more regular and consistent the contractions. Endorphins

are natural substances released by the body under stress. They have three main purposes: to modify pain, alter perception of time and space, and encourage well-being. Once labour begins, endorphin levels rise to help you to cope with painful contractions. If you are fearful, adrenaline will inhibit oxytocin and endorphin production.

NATURAL PAIN RELIEF

There are natural methods of pain relief that can be used as alternatives to conventional means such as anaesthetics

(for example, an epidural), inhaled analgesics (gas and air) or narcotics (pethidine).

• **Acupuncture** A qualified practitioner can help to relieve pain, boost energy levels and encourage you to control fear. Needles inserted into acupoints in the ear can be attached to an electro-acupuncture, or acutens, machine to stimulate the release of endorphins. You control the level of stimulation. You will feel a warm thudding sensation in your ear. It takes 30–40 minutes to build up the endorphin level enough to ease

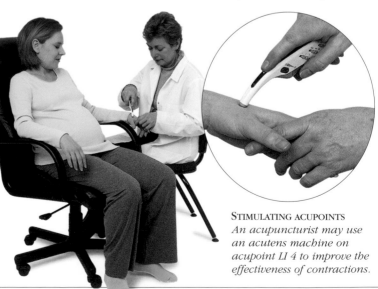

STIMULATING ACUPOINTS
An acupuncturist may use an acutens machine on acupoint LI 4 to improve the effectiveness of contractions.

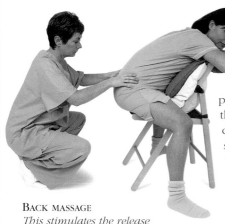

BACK MASSAGE
This stimulates the release of endorphins, the body's natural pain-killers.

painful contractions. To relieve backache, an acupuncturist will insert needles into acupoints Bl 31 and Bl 32 in the sacral region of the lower spine, or your partner can apply pressure. A TENS machine (*see page 109*) can also be used. This blocks pain receptors and is useful in early labour. Abdominal pain may be eased by treating acupoints Liv 3 (between the first and second toes) and GB 34 (outside leg just below the knee) to relax muscles and tendons. Acupuncture can also be used to improve weak or slow contractions by boosting the flow of *qi*. Again, Bl 31 and Bl 32 are the acupoints used.

• **Homeopathy** Remedies for pain relief include *Aconite 6c*, for contractions that occur in rapid succession with acute back pain; *Pulsatilla 6c*, for backache that is cutting and spasmodic; and *Belladonna 6c*, when pain extends from the back down the thighs. For abdominal pain try *Chamomilla 6c*, for spasmodic pain; and *Gelsemium 6c*, for cramps.

• **Massage** This is one of the simplest and most time-honoured ways of relieving pain. It helps to decrease the intensity of pain by dissipating tension. Massage should be rhythmical but varied, using different pressures and speeds. In general, a slow massage will calm and a brisk one will stimulate. Firm but gentle strokes using the flat of the hand and stroking towards the heart will ease tension. This should be done for at least 20 minutes to encourage endorphins to be released. Using the appropriate essential oil may be beneficial: lavender for relief of pain; mandarin to lift the spirits; and clary sage to improve contractions in an attempt to speed up a painful, protracted labour. Clary sage is a potent oil, however, and should

be pre-prepared by and used under strict instruction of a practitioner. Other suitable oils include chamomile, eucalyptus and frankincense.

OTHER USEFUL THERAPIES

• **Reflexology** Reflex points on the ankle bones correspond to the uterus and pelvic region. These can be stimulated in order to relieve pain and stress and to regulate contractions.
• **Hypnosis** Techniques of self-hypnosis to help you to control pain can be learnt beforehand.
• **Yoga** Regular yoga practice will put you in tune with your body so that you understand its natural responses during labour rather than resisting them and possibly losing control.

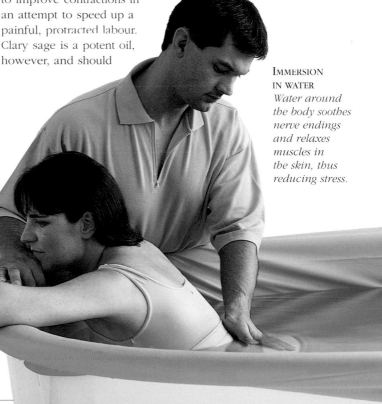

**IMMERSION
IN WATER**
Water around the body soothes nerve endings and relaxes muscles in the skin, thus reducing stress.

Inducing Labour

INDUCTION IS A DELIBERATE attempt to start labour by artificial means. Most women would prefer to go into labour naturally, but the safety of mother and baby is paramount. In certain circumstances the risk of continuing a pregnancy is greater than the potential risk of intervention by means of induction.

REASONS FOR INDUCTION

Rates of induction vary from hospital to hospital and from consultant to consultant. Find out what the induction policy is at your hospital so that you know what to expect if it is necessary. Induction may be recommended if:

• The baby has gone more than seven days beyond term (maximum 14 days). The danger is that the placenta will start to fail and the baby will lack oxygen. You may be asked to monitor the baby's activity.

• Your blood pressure is raised. Induction will depend upon the severity of your condition, the amount of protein in your urine and the maturity of the baby.

• You have gestational diabetes. This may put the baby at risk in late pregnancy. Induction may be recommended at about 37 weeks if there are indications that the baby is unwell.

• The membranes rupture early. Some hospitals advise induction, while others check that the umbilical cord has not come down and send you home to wait for labour to start.

• You have a poor obstetric history, for example placental abruption (placenta starts coming away from the uterine wall), stillbirth or foetal abnormality. A growing number of women want to know exactly when their baby will be born and request induction. It carries a risk, however, and should only be done for medical reasons.

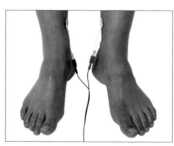

USING A **TENS** MACHINE
Attach a TENS machine (see page 109) to Sp 6 on each inside leg, four fingers' width above the ankle, to start induction.

METHODS OF INDUCTION

The following methods or products may be used.

• Sweeping the membranes. This can be done as part of a vaginal examination. It may be a little painful but can induce labour if you are close to term.

• Prostaglandin gel. Pessaries containing this hormone are inserted into the vagina, or gel is applied around the cervix (unless the membranes have ruptured), to ripen the cervix and stimulate contractions.

• Intravenous oxytocin. You will be put on a drip of this drug to initiate contractions.

NATURAL ALTERNATIVES

If labour begins spontaneously, contractions build up gradually. Endorphins are released to help you to cope with the build-up of pain. If you are induced, this natural process is short-circuited. The pain comes fast and can be acute. Without the chance to prepare, many women lose control and demand pain relief. You will usually be given several days' notice of an induction, which gives you the opportunity to try natural alternatives. Only do this if your pregnancy has been free of complications and you are at term. Consult your midwife first.

• **Acupuncture** Needles will be inserted into acupoints on the back. Two or three sessions over a week may be necessary. Also try acupressure or a TENS machine on LI 4 and Sp 6.

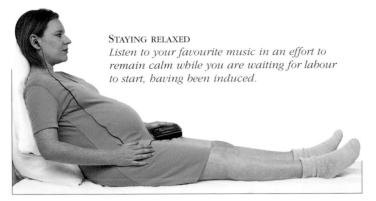

- **Homeopathy** Take *Secale
30c* or *Caulophyllum 30c* (as
directed by a practitioner)
until your contractions start.
Caulophyllum should not be
used if you have a history
of quick labour.
- **Reflexology** Treatment
will be applied to the pituitary
reflexes. It is advisable to
consult a qualified practitioner.
- **Cranial osteopathy** This may
stimulate the pituitary gland
to produce the hormones
that are important for labour.
- **Herbalism** Drink raspberry
leaf tea four times a day.

COPING WITH INDUCTION

Once labour is underway,
you may well need some help
in dealing with contractions.
- **Acupressure**. With advice
from a practitioner beforehand,
mark the relevant acupoints on
your body and apply a TENS
machine (*see page 109*) to
stimulate them or get your
partner to massage them if
the pain is severe. Use Bl 31
and Bl 32 in the sacral region
of the lower back for back
pain and Sp 8 on the inside
lower leg for abdominal
pain. Alternatively, take an
acupuncturist with you into
the delivery room.

- **Flower remedies** A few
drops directly on the tongue
or added to a glass of water
may help you to cope as labour
progresses. Take Five Flower
Formula or Rescue Remedy for
panic, shock or fear; cherry
plum if you are at the end of
your tether; gorse if you feel
hopeless and that your labour
is endless; and rock rose for
fear and panic.
- **Homeopathy** A homeopath
may attend the birth or give
advice over the phone, having
prepared various remedies for
you in advance. These might
include *Aconite 6c*, for severe,
rapid contractions, soreness
in the back and fear;
Chamomilla 6c, for

PROVIDING SUPPORT
*Pain can come fast and
strong. In this position
a partner can
provide support
as well as
reassurance.*

unbearable, spasmodic
contractions, back pain and
oversensitivity to noise and
pain; *Cimic. 6c*, for severe
contractions, a bruised feeling,
restlessness, irritability and
chilliness; *Coffea 6c*, for severe
back pain and the urge to bear
down before the cervix is fully
dilated; *Secale cornutum 6c*, for
irregular, ineffectual contractions
that are causing distress.
- **Aromatherapy** For backache,
massage with lavender, clary
sage (under direction by a
practitioner) or chamomile
oils diluted in a carrier oil; for
encouraging contractions and
labour, lavender, clary sage,
jasmine or rose; to refresh and
revitalize, a drop of lemon,
lime or grapefruit placed in the
palm of the hand; for hysteria,
a drop of frankincense placed
in the palm of the hand.

First Stage of Labour

ACQUAINTING YOURSELF WITH THE DIFFERENT STAGES and behaviour patterns of labour is useful preparation for the event and will help you greatly when the time comes, especially if you are apprehensive or even fearful. In addition, there is a wealth of gentle, complementary remedies to assist you in labour.

WHAT HAPPENS

The length of the first stage of labour with a first baby is on average 12–14 hours (less in subsequent pregnancies). The cervix opens gradually, dilating to 10 cm at the rate of approximately 1 cm an hour. The baby moves down into the pelvis, gradually turning so that it is facing is your back.

THE ROLE OF YOUR MIDWIFE

A midwife's job is to keep an eye on both you and the baby, checking the progress of your labour. Initially she will palpate your abdomen gently to see how the baby is lying and how far the head is engaged. She will note your temperature, pulse rate, blood pressure and any swelling of the ankles. She will listen to the baby's heartbeat, which should be strong and regular (110–150 beats a minute). You may be attached to a cardiotachograph (CTG) machine, which monitors contractions and the baby's heartbeat. Every 4–5 hours your

midwife will give you a vaginal examination to assess how far the cervix has dilated.

THE BABY'S POSITION

The way the baby is lying at the end of your pregnancy will have a significant effect on the kind of labour you are likely to have. The most favourable position is with the baby's back facing your front: the occipital anterior position. Many babies today, especially with first-time mothers and often as a result of a sedentary lifestyle, present in the occipital posterior position, with the baby's back facing your back. The baby will turn

during delivery, but this may prolong your labour (*see page 109*, Coping with *Induction, for dealing with a difficult labour*). To help the baby get into position in the final weeks of pregnancy, avoid sitting cross-legged; stand leaning forward against a wall for 10–20 minutes twice a day in the last six weeks; avoid reclining positions, such as sitting slumped on a sofa; and go swimming and practise yoga, which are helpful forms of gentle exercise.

EARLY LABOUR

As the cervix dilates from 0 cm to 4 cm try to conserve energy but keep mobile, using gravity to help the baby's head to descend and press on the cervix, keeping contractions going. If necessary, squat or sit on a chair during contractions. If you

TAKING UP POSITIONS
Your midwife will help you to relax into positions that help your labour to progress and ensure that you breathe correctly.

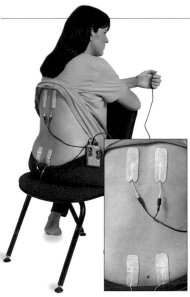

TENS MACHINE
*Pads are easily attached to
specific points on the back
to block pain messages.*

have back pain, kneel on
all fours and ask your partner
to massage your back. This
position will help the pelvis
to open: also try rocking the
pelvis. Develop your own
pattern of breathing, slowly to
keep calm, faster as the body
requires more oxygen.

ACCELERATED PHASE

Once labour is established,
the contractions will speed up,
occurring every 2–3 minutes,
lasting 45–60 seconds, and
feeling stronger and more
intense. During this phase,
your cervix will dilate from
4 cm to 8 cm. This is a good
time to get into a birthing pool
or bath. You will want to rest
between contractions by now,
finding the most comfortable
position and supported by your
partner or midwife and by
pillows and cushions. It may be
difficult to get comfortable and
your partner's support will be

vitally important. You will have
lost your appetite but you will
be thirsty. You may become
withdrawn, avoiding eye contact
and conversation. Your partner
should be aware that you will
not want noise or disruption.
Try the following remedies
and methods of pain relief.
• Use a TENS (Transcutaneous
Electrical Nerve Stimulation)
machine (*see left*). Electrodes
in pads are attached to specific
points on the back. A pulsed
electric current blocks pain
messages from the cervix and
uterus to the brain. A control
box allows you to alter the
intensity of the current. A TENS
machine can be bought or hired
a few weeks before the birth.
• Try to identify the location
of pain and the nature of other
problems, such as slow or
ineffectual contractions, and
use the appropriate remedies
(*see pages 102–3*).
• Take Rescue Remedy or
mimulus flower remedy if you
are feeling fearful or panicky.
• Use essential oils of lavender,
frankincense, mandarin and
chamomile to help to relieve
anxiety or stress. Massage a
drop of whichever you like
into the plam of your hand
to release the aroma.
• If you feel nauseous, sniff
peppermint essential oil.
• Take *Pulsatilla 6c* (dosage:
every 20 minutes for up to
seven doses) if you feel weepy,
you keep apologising and your
mood is very changeable.
• Try to maintain positions that
help to tilt your pelvis forward
and encourage the baby into
the most desirable position for
the birth, open up the pelvic

outlet and keep contractions
going (*see opposite, below and
see also pages 74–5*).

TRANSITION

This is often the most difficult
part of labour, as the cervix
dilates to 10 cm (4 in) and
the opening out phase changes
to the bearing down phase.
Contractions will be at their
strongest, 1–3½ minutes
apart and lasting 45–90
seconds. It will be
hard to stay in
control: you may
feel nauseous,
shivery, irritable
and anxious. Take
Rescue Remedy and
star of Bethlehem
flower remedy
if you are
struggling. Some
women prefer
to get out of a
birthing pool
at this stage.

**KEEPING
UPRIGHT**
*Encourage the
baby's head to
descend and
keep contractions
going by being
upright. Rest
by leaning
against a wall
for support with
knees bent slightly.*

Second Stage of Labour

THE SECOND STAGE OF LABOUR is the period from full dilation of the cervix to the birth. On average, this lasts about an hour in a first pregnancy but less in subsequent ones. With a renewed burst of energy, you will develop a strong and irresistible urge to push the baby down the birth canal.

KEY TIPS

Take your time, do not feel rushed and rest between pushes

✳

Get your partner to sponge your face and neck

✳

Take sips of iced water

HOW YOU WILL FEEL

The transition phase brings a surge of endorphins before the urge to push signals the start of the second stage. You may feel calmer, with a renewed sense of focus and purpose. You will begin to feel more passive, less active. Find a position that is comfortable. Try squatting, supported by your partner, on all fours or over a bean bag, or kneeling on a bed. Once the cervix is fully dilated, the pain feels like cramp or a burning sensation. Contractions will be shorter and further apart. Your

waters will break if they have not already done so. The urge to push builds gradually. Follow this urge as it suits you: do what your body feels it has to.

USING REMEDIES

Complentary remedies may be useful in the second stage.
• Apply gentle pressure to acupoints GB 21, at the top of the shoulder near the neck, or LI 4, between the forefinger and thumb to stimulate contractions if they are infrequent or the gap between them lengthens.

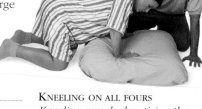

KNEELING ON ALL FOURS
Kneeling may be less tiring than other positions. Keep your back straight and relax forwards on to a cushion between contractions.

• Homeopathic remedies include: *Coffea 6c* if you are despairing, with no urge to push; *Kali carb. 6c* if you have become obstinate and dilation has ceased; *Secale 6c* if you are distressed and want to push.
• Mugwort flower remedy promotes birthing, five flower formula will help you stay calm and centred and walnut may help you to adjust to the rapid physical changes.
• Essential oils of lemon, lime, grapefruit, mandarin, jasmine or rose – vapourized or used for gentle massage – will lift mood.

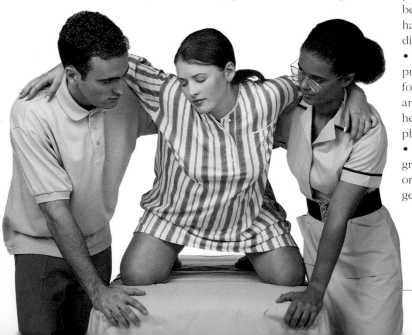

POSITION FOR DELIVERY
Kneeling is a good position from which to push. Your midwife and partner can support you.

Third Stage of Labour

THE THIRD STAGE OF LABOUR follows the birth and lasts about 30 minutes. During this time the "afterbirth" (placenta and membranes) is delivered, but you will be concentrating on your new baby. You may well be feeling euphoric, with a strong urge to bond as you hold your baby to your breast.

THE BIRTH

As the baby is born, your midwife will control its passage through the vagina so as to minimize the risk of tearing the perineum. Once the head has been born, the shoulders and the rest of the body quickly follow and your baby is delivered on to your stomach. As the baby's shoulder is presented, you may be given an injection of a drug called syntometrine. This makes the womb contract and expel the placenta quickly, thus preventing excessive bleeding. This is known as active management of the third stage. It does carry a small risk of minor side effects to you and the baby. Discuss with your midwife whether or not you want this. Your attention will by now, however, be entirely focused on your new baby, and you will have few memories of the physical sensations of the third stage. Endorphins released during the birth promote a euphoric state and strengthen the natural urge to bond. You may feel elated, with a strong instinct to sit up and gather your baby to the breast.

USING NATURAL REMEDIES

These can be used for several purposes after the birth.
• For a retained placenta, apply pressure to acupoints CV 4 on the lower abdomen, Bl 67 on the little toe nail, or GB 21 in the shoulder "well". Alternatively, massage the abdomen with diluted clary sage oil, take the homeopathic remedy *Caulophyllum 6c* or mugwort flower remedy to encourage uterine contractions.
• To relieve after pains, shock, soft-tissue damage, soreness, swelling and bruising, take *Arnica 6c*. Also for shock, try *Aconite 6c* or Rescue Remedy or Five Flower Formula.

BONDING WITH YOUR BABY
It is natural to put a baby to the breast soon after the birth. This releases oxytocin, which helps the placenta to come away.

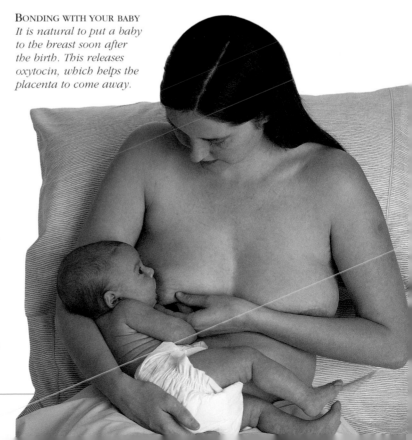

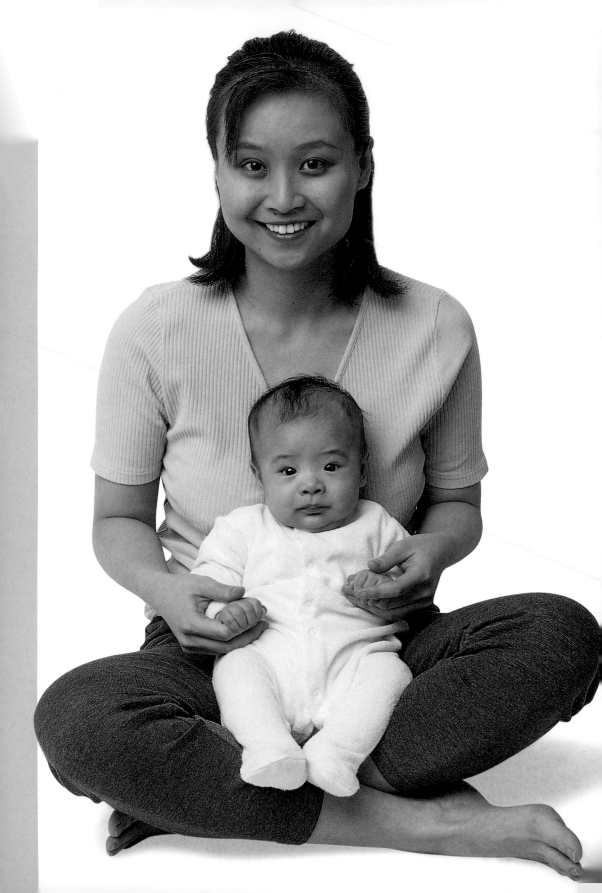